Manfred Georg Krukemeyer and Gunnar Moellenhoff (Eds.)

Endoprosthetics

Endoprosthetics

An Introduction for the Practitioner

Edited by
Manfred Georg Krukemeyer and Gunnar Moellenhoff

DE GRUYTER

Editors

Manfred Georg Krukemeyer, M.D.
Paracelsus-Kliniken
Sedanstrasse 109
49076 Osnabrueck, Germany
e-mail: dr-krukemeyer@t-online.de

Gunnar Moellenhoff, M.D., Professor of Orthopedic Surgery
Department of Trauma Surgery and Orthopedic Surgery
Raphaelsklinik Muenster GmbH
Loerstrasse 23
48143 Muenster, Germany
e-mail: g.moellenhoff@raphaelsklinik.de

ISBN 978-3-11-030510-4
e-ISBN 978-3-11-030513-5

Library of Congress Cataloging-in-Publication Data
A CIP catalog record for this book has been applied for at the Library of Congress.

Bibliographic information published by the Deutsche Nationalbibliothek
The Deutsche Nationalbibliothek lists this publication in the Deutsche Nationalbibliografie; detailed bibliographic data are available in the Internet at http://dnb.dnb.de.

Typesetting: Meta Systems Publishing & Printservices GmbH, Wustermark
Printing and binding: Hubert & Co. GmbH und Co. KG, Göttingen
♾ Printed on acid-free paper
Printed in Germany

www.degruyter.com

Preface

After submitting the third edition of their book “Endoprosthetics” in German, the editors were asked to publish an English-language version.

In the Western world, the field of endoprosthetics is demonstrating rapid growth. Due to the aging of the population in Western society, the use of endoprosthetic treatments – such as the replacement of injured or damaged joints with artificial joints – is in ever greater demand. Reliable long-term clinical results are achievable using specific indicators and a meticulous approach.

This textbook includes chapters on important topics, such as (unknown until only a few years ago) the minimally-invasive techniques of endoprosthetics, tumor endoprosthetics and complications resulting in the revision of endoprosthetics.

The authors and publishers have completely revised this version for the English-speaking market. In developing the concept of the English-language edition, we have focused on the most important topics. As in other medical fields, the technique of implantation and the material of endoprosthesis are constantly evolving – new information has been added and out-of-date material deleted.

We thank Walter de Gruyter publishers for proofreading, translation and the successful publication of this book. We would like to wish the readers enjoyable reading and would be grateful for any suggestions or comments.

Muenster, Germany 2013

Manfred Georg Krukemeyer and
Gunnar Moellenhoff

List of contributing authors

Editors

Manfred Georg Krukemeyer, M.D.
Paracelsus-Kliniken
Sedanstrasse 109
49076 Osnabrueck, Germany

Gunnar Moellenhoff, M.D.,
Professor of Orthopedic Surgery
Department of Trauma Surgery and
Orthopedic Surgery
Raphaelsklinik Muenster GmbH
Loerstrasse 23
48143 Muenster, Germany

Authors

Peter Aldinger, M.D.,
Professor of Orthopedic Surgery
Orthopedic Clinic Paulinenhilfe
Diakonie Klinikum Stuttgart
Rosenbergstrasse 38
70176 Stuttgart, Germany

Georg Gosheger, M.D.,
Professor of Orthopedic Surgery
Tumor Orthopedics and
Revision Endoprosthetics
Clinic for General Orthopedics and
Tumor Orthopedics
University Medical Center Muenster
Albert-Schweitzer-Campus 1
48149 Muenster, Germany

Jendrik Hardes, M.D.,
Professor of Orthopedic Surgery
Tumor Orthopedics and
Revision Endoprosthetics
Clinic for General Orthopedics and
Tumor Orthopedics
University Medical Center Muenster
Albert-Schweitzer-Campus 1
48149 Muenster, Germany

Joachim Herre, M.D.
Orthopedic Clinic Paulinenhilfe
Diakonie Klinikum Stuttgart
Rosenbergstrasse 38
70176 Stuttgart, Germany

Steffen Hoell, M.D.
Tumor Orthopedics and
Revision Endoprosthetics
Clinic for General Orthopedics and
Tumor Orthopedics
University Medical Center Muenster
Albert-Schweitzer-Campus 1
48149 Muenster, Germany

Robert Hube, M.D.
Orthopedic Surgery Munich (OCM)
Steinerstrasse 6
81369 Munich, Germany

Michael John, M.D.
Clinical Centre of Trauma Surgery and Orthopedics
Clinic for Orthopedics
Clinical Center Magdeburg gGmbH
Birkenallee 34
39130 Magdeburg, Germany

Hartmuth Kiefer, M.D.,
Professor of Orthopedic Surgery
Department of Trauma Surgery and
Orthopedic Surgery, Hand and Restoration Surgery
Lukas-Krankenhaus Bünde
Akademisches Lehrkrankenhaus der MH Hannover
Hindenburgstrasse 56
32257 Buende, Germany

Olaf Kilian, M.D., Professor of Surgery
Zentralklinik Bad Berka GmbH
Robert-Koch-Allee 9
99437 Bad Berka, Germany

Sebastian Lieske, M.D.
Clinical Centre of Trauma Surgery and Orthopedics
Clinic for Orthopedics
Clinical Center Magdeburg gGmbH
Birkenallee 34
39130 Magdeburg, Germany

Bjoern Marquardt, M.D.
Orthopedic Surgery
Von-Vincke-Strasse 14
48143 Muenster, Germany

Christian Merle, M.D.
Clinical Centre of Trauma Surgery and Orthopedics
University Clinic Heidelberg
Schlierbacher Landstrasse 200a
69118 Heidelberg, Germany

Hans-Wolfram Neumann, M.D.
Professor of Orthopedic Surgery
Orthopedic University Hospital
Otto von Guericke University Magdeburg
Leipziger Strasse 44
39112 Magdeburg, Germany

Markus Nottrott, M.D.
Tumor Orthopedics and Revision Endoprosthetics
Clinic for General Orthopedics and
Tumor Orthopedics
University Medical Center Muenster
Albert-Schweitzer-Campus 1
48149 Muenster, Germany

Katja Schenk, M.D.
Orthopedic University Hospital
Otto von Guericke University Magdeburg
Leipziger Strasse 44
39112 Magdeburg, Germany

Iris Schleicher, M.D.
Clinic and Polyclinic of Trauma Surgery
University Clinic Giessen and Marburg
Rudolf-Buchheim-Strasse 7
35385 Gießen, Germany

Reinhard Schnettler, M.D., Professor of Surgery
Clinic and Polyclinic of Trauma Surgery
University Clinic Giessen and Marburg
Rudolf-Buchheim-Strasse 7
35385 Gießen, Germany

Dominik Schorn, M.D.
Department of Trauma Surgery
and Orthopedic Surgery
Raphaelsklinik Muenster GmbH
Loerstraße 23
48143 Muenster, Germany

Joern Steinbeck, M.D.,
Professor of Orthopedic Surgery
Orthopedic Surgery
Von-Vincke-Strasse 14
48143 Muenster, Germany

Arne Streitbuerger, M.D.
Tumor Orthopedics and Revision Endoprosthetics
Clinic for General Orthopedics and
Tumor Orthopedics
University Medical Center Muenster
Albert-Schweitzer-Campus 1
48149 Muenster, Germany

Kai-Axel Witt, M.D.
Orthopedic Surgery
Von-Vincke-Straße 14
48143 Muenster, Germany

Contents

Abbreviations

a.p.	anterior–posterior
AAOS	American Academy of Orthopedic Surgeons
ACL	anterior cruciate ligament
ADL	activity of daily living
AE	Arbeitsgemeinschaft Endoprothetik {German organization for endoprosthetics}
ASIS	anterior spina iliaca superior
BHR	Birmingham Hip Resurfacing
BMI	body mass index
BMP	bone morphogenic proteins
BSG	Blutsenkungsgeschwindigkeit {erythrocyte sedimentation rate = ESR}
BW	body weight
BWR	Bewertungsrelation {cost weight = CW}
CAD	coronary artery disease
CAS	computer-assisted surgery
CCD	caput-collum-diaphyseal angle
CCL	complication and co-morbidity level
CFK	carbon-faserverstärkter Kunststoff {carbon-fiber-reinforced plastic = CFRP}
CFU	colony-forming unit
COPD	chronic obstructive pulmonary disease
CPM	continuous passive motion
CRP	C-reactive protein
CT	computed tomography
d	day
DLC	diamond-like carbon
DmpT	N,N-Dimethyl-p-toluidine
DRG	diagnosis-related groups
DSA	digital subtraction angiography
DVT	deep vein thrombosis
EAP	extended ambulant rehabilitation
EFORT	European Federation of National Associations of Orthopaedics and Traumatology
EPRD	Endoprosthesenregister Deutschlands {German endoprosthesis register}
FDA	Federal Food and Drug Administration
FFP	fresh frozen plasma
HA	hydroxyapatite
HE	hematoxylin–eosin
HIT	heparin-induced thrombocytopenia
HO	heterotopic ossification
HPF	high-power field
ICC	intraclass correlation coefficient
ICF	International Classification of Functioning, Disability and Health
IL-10	interleukin-10
IL-6	interleukin-6
InEK	Institut für das Entgeltsystem im Krankenhaus GmbH {Institute for the *Hospital* Remuneration System}
IRO	internal rotation
KHEntgG	Krankenhausentgeltgesetz {Hospital Remuneration Law}
LE	lung embolism

LISS	less invasive stabilization system
LMWH	low-molecular-weight heparin
LPS	lipopolysaccharide
M.	musculus, muscle
MDC	major diagnosis category
MIS	minimally invasive surgery
MOM	metal-on-metal
MRSA	methicillin-resistant Staphylococcus aureus
MRSE	methicillin-resistant Staphylococcus epidermidis
MRT	magnetic resonance tomography
MSTS	Musculoskeletal Tumor Society
NPV	negative predictive value
NRS	numeric rating scale
NSAID	non-steroidal anti-inflammatory drugs
OATS	osteochondral autologous transplantation
OPS	Operation and Procedures Key {For medical insurance claims}
p.a.	posterior–anterior
p.o.	postoperative
PACS	picture and archiving and communication system
PAOD	peripheral artery occlusive disease
PAS	*Periodic* acid–*Schiff stain*
PCA	patient-controlled anesthesia
PCCL	patient clinical complexity level
PCL	posterior cruciate ligament = PCL
PCT	procalcitonin
PDC	peridural catheter
PDGF	platelet-derived growth factor
PE	polyethylene
PET	polyethylene terephthalate
PET	positron emission tomography
PIR	post-isometric relaxation
PMMA	polymethyl methacrylate
PNF	proprioceptive neuromuscular facilitation
PPV	positive predictive value
PVNS	pigmented villomodular synovitis
RKI	Robert Koch Institute
ROM	range of motion/movement
SCV	small colony variants
TEP	total endoprosthesis
TGF	transforming growth factor
TNFα	tumor necrosis factor α
TPP	thrust plate prosthesis = TPP
UHMWPE	ultra-high-molecular-weight polyethylene
VAS	visual analog scale
VRE	vancomycin-resistant enterococci
WHO	World Health Organization
WOMAC	Western Ontario and MacMasters Universities Osteoarthritis Index
X-PE	cross-linked polyethylene

D. Schorn, B. Marquardt, K.-A. Witt, J. Steinbeck

1 Shoulder Endoprosthetics

1.1 Introduction

After the introduction of the prototype of a shoulder prosthesis by Charles Neer in the 1950s, shoulder endoprosthetics gained increasing significance in orthopedic surgery. Thus, in 2007 approximately 10,000 implantations were carried out, with an upward trend and patient satisfaction of 80 % (hemiprosthesis) up to 90 % (total endoprosthesis). The technical concepts of the implants used were guided by the original anatomy of the healthy shoulder and were aimed at reproducing this as accurately as possible. The increasing understanding of the relevant anatomy of the shoulder joint led to a steady development of shoulder endoprostheses that even today is not over. Moreover, the spectrum of indications for shoulder endoprosthetics has increasingly expanded and has led to the development of special prostheses such as a cap prosthesis, the reverse shoulder prosthesis or the resurfacing or partial resurfacing.

Shoulder endoprostheses:
- Approximately 10,000 a year
- 80–90 % patient satisfaction
- Orientation to the anatomy of the healthy shoulder
- Reconstruction of the original anatomy

1.2 History and Development of Shoulder Endoprosthetics

Modern shoulder endoprosthetics were established in the 1950s by Charles Neer. The so-called Neer mark I prosthesis was an unlinked fracture prosthesis, which was primarily conceived for the treatment of humeral head breaks.

Neer prosthesis series I:
Fracture prosthesis for the treatment of humeral head fractures

In 1973, this prosthesis was modified to become the Neer mark II prosthesis. As a non-modular monoblock prosthesis, it was regarded as a typical representative of the so-called first-generation shoulder prostheses (Fig. 1.1). For many years it was also seen to be the standard prosthesis, because, owing to the various sheath lengths and thicknesses, as well as different sizes of the integrated prosthesis head, for the first time more individual customization was possible. At the same time the prosthesis was complemented by the possibility of a glenoid replacement. This was a glenoid component made of polyethylene with a radius that fitted the humerus head and "keel" component to the cemented implantation. However, a complete replication of the individual ball anatomy was not possible with the Neer mark II prosthesis either.

Neer prosthesis mark II:
- First-generation shoulder prostheses
- Long standard prosthesis
- Non-modular monoblock prosthesis

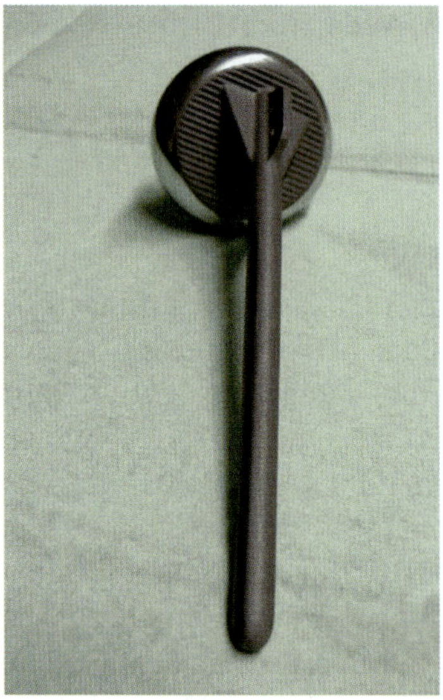

Fig. 1.1: Neer series II monoblock prosthesis.

Second-generation shoulder prostheses with the concept of modularity

With the second-generation prostheses at the end of the 1980s the concept of modularity found its way into shoulder endoprosthetics. Different stems could be combined with various balls with a metal cone joint.

An anatomically correct reconstruction of the centre of rotation was, however, not possible with first- and second-generation prostheses. A modified, unphysiological socket load was the conse-

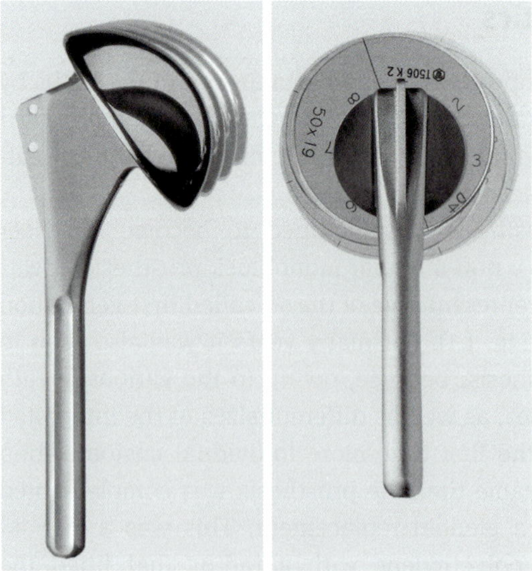

(a) (b)

Fig. 1.2: (a, b) Conventional third-generation modular sheath prosthesis (Aequalis, Tornier).

quence. This difficulty led to the Aequalis prosthesis (Tornier) (Fig. 1.2). As a typical representative of third-generation shoulder prostheses this implant permitted biaxial adjustability, i.e., head eccentricity, and the humeral angle of inclination was variably adjustable, so that the prosthesis could be adapted to the head anatomy.

Third-generation shoulder prostheses: biaxial adjustability possible

To guarantee smooth modularity in three axes it was also necessary to release the version of the prosthesis head, i.e., the link between the stem of the prosthesis and the ball. This three-dimensional variability is provided by prosthesis models conceived by von Habermeyer (Univers/Arthrex) and Gerber (Anatomica/Zimmer) among others of the fourth generation (Fig. 1.3).

Fourth-generation shoulder prostheses: smooth modularity on three axes

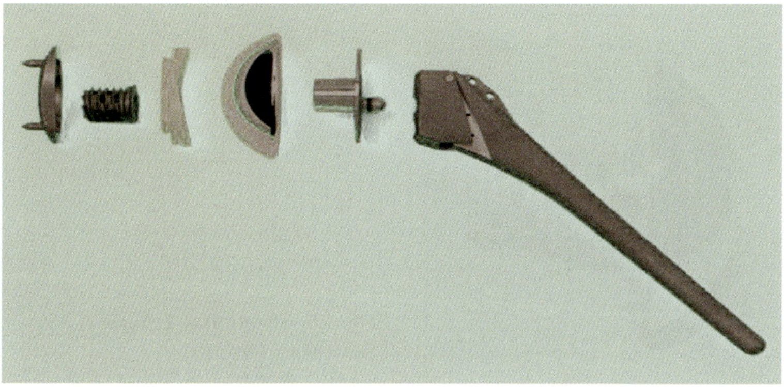

Fig. 1.3: Fourth-generation Univers 3D prosthesis (Arthrex).

Unlike with the conventional stem prosthesis, the concept of endoprosthetic resurfacing at the shoulder joint mainly affects only the replacement of the destroyed joint surface with reproduction of the normal anatomy with minimal bone resection. The so-called cap prostheses were originally developed for the treatment of rheumatoid arthritis of the shoulder at the beginning of the 1980s in

Surface replacement (cap prosthesis): replacement of the destroyed joint surface, reproduction of the normal anatomy with minimal bone resection

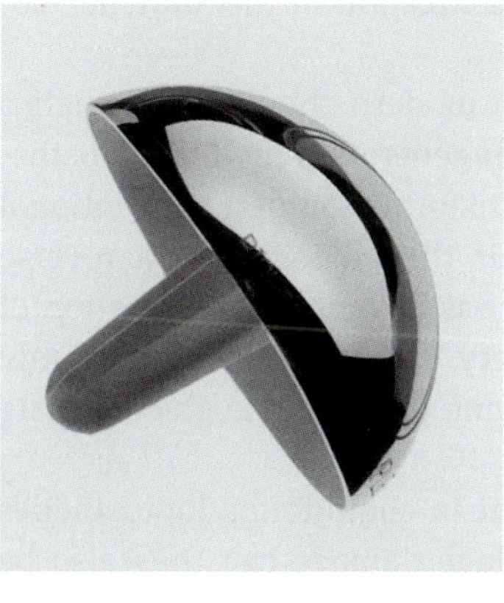

Fig. 1.4: Copeland cup (Biomet).

In 2006 approximately 1,500 surface replacements/10,000 shoulder prosthesis implants

Stem-free humeral cap prostheses with minimal bone resection

Sweden. Humeral resurfacing was popularized by Copeland in England after he also extended the indications to shoulder arthrosis (Fig. 1.4). According to industry data, out of approximately 10,000 implanted shoulder prostheses, about 1,500 were cancelled in favor of resurfacing implants in Germany in 2006.

The concept of minimal bone resection continued with new stem-free humeral cap prostheses such as the Eclipse prosthesis (Arthrex) (Fig. 1.5), in which not only the cartilage is removed up to the subchondral bone, but the whole humeral head along the anatomical neck is resected. A considerable advantage of this prosthesis model in comparison to the conventional cap prosthesis is the distinctly simplified access to the glenoid.

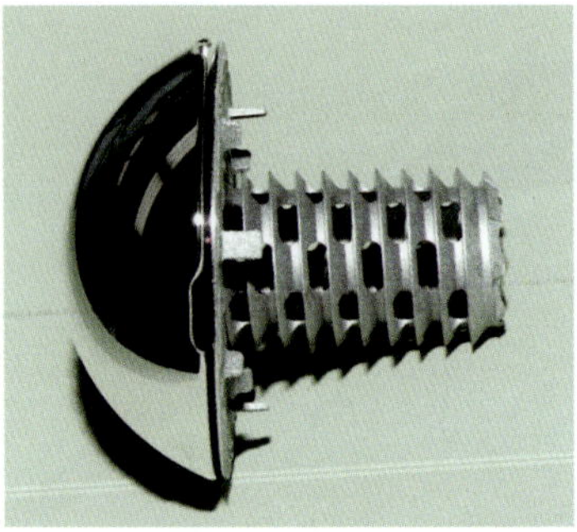

Fig. 1.5: Sheath-free Eclipse prosthesis (Arthrex).

Delta Mark III prosthesis:
- Prototype of the reverse prosthesis
- Concept: rotation of the anatomical relationship between the glenoid and humeral components
- Good mobility with low luxation tendency

An additional benefit of modern shoulder prosthetics was the development of the reverse shoulder prosthesis (Fig. 1.6). Contrary to the prosthesis designs described so far, the concept involved in the reverse prosthesis is based upon a reversal of the anatomical relationship between the glenoid and humeral components and is especially effective in the presence of a pronounced rotator cuff injury. A prototype of the modern reverse prosthesis is the Delta III prosthesis developed by Paul Grammont (Depuy), which achieves through medialization and caudalization of the center of rotation extensive mobility with a low tendency toward luxation in this difficult biomechanical location.

Fifth generation of shoulder prostheses: enables transformation of a conventional shoulder prosthesis with or without the glenoid in reverse shoulder prosthesis

The most recent development in modern shoulder prosthetics is demonstrated by the so-called fifth-generation modular prostheses, which if required enable the transformation of a conventional shoulder prosthesis with or without the glenoid into a reverse shoulder prosthesis (Fig. 1.7). If there is advanced degeneration of the rotator cuff such revision surgery can be made significantly easier; the prosthesis stem and in some products the glenoid plate can be retained as well.

Another very recent development in shoulder endoprosthetics is partial resurfacing. Isolated cartilage damage can thus also be

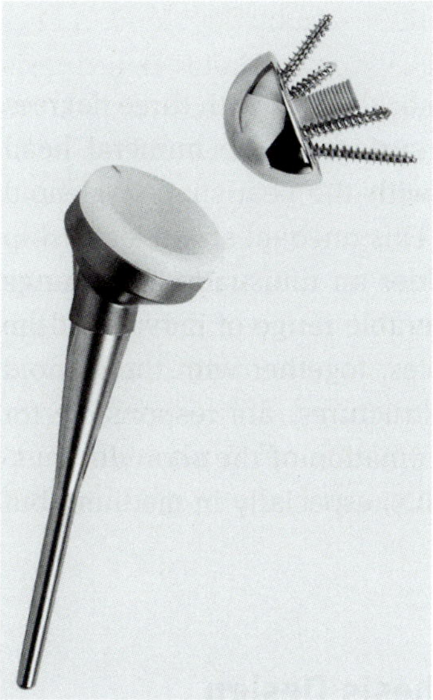

Fig. 1.6: Inverse prosthesis (Aequalis Reversed, Tornier).

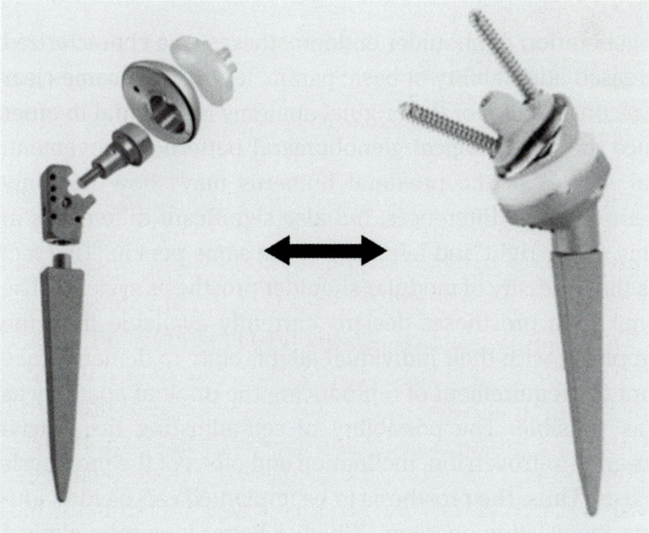

Fig. 1.7: Fifth-generation modular, convertible shoulder prosthesis (Promos, Smith & Nephew).

specifically addressed without affecting the intact cartilage surface. Here, with the Partial Eclipse, Arthrex has developed a partial resurfacing component that can be inserted arthroscopically and thus without removal of the subscapularis muscle. However, long-term results for partial resurfacing in shoulder endoprosthetics are not yet available.

Partial surface replacement:
targeted addressing of isolated cartilage damage without affecting the intact cartilage surface

1.3 Anatomy

Anatomy of the shoulder joint

The glenohumeral joint is a ball and socket joint with three degrees of freedom, by which the articular surface of the humeral head (approximately 0.24 m^2) articulates with the pear-shaped glenoid cavity of the scapula (only 0.06 m^2). This unequal size relationship of the joint surfaces gives the shoulder an unusually large range of movement. In spite of this considerable range of movement the joint remains stable. The joint surfaces, together with the glenoid labrum and the capsular ligament structures, are responsible for the static stability. The complex coordination of the shoulder musculature brings about dynamic stability, especially in medium, but also terminal range of movement.

1.4 Biomechanics and Prosthesis Design

1.4.1 Humeral Head Prosthesis

Exact reconstruction of the original anatomy is essential for the reproduction of the physiological glenohumeral pattern of movement

Each new generation of shoulder endoprostheses was characterized by the increased adaptability of basic parameters, as it became clear that exact reconstruction of the original anatomy is essential in order to reproduce the physiological glenohumeral pattern of movement. Anatomical studies of the proximal humerus may show not only strong interindividual differences, but also significant differences in the anatomy of the right and left sides of the same person. This fact underlines the necessity of modular shoulder prosthesis systems. The conventional stem prostheses designs currently available from the various suppliers, with their individual adaptability to demand, take into account the requirement of reproducing the original anatomy as precisely as possible. The possibility of self-adjusting the crucial parameters ante-/retroversion, inclination and offset of the prosthesis (Fig. 1.2) exists. Thus, the prosthesis to be implanted can be individually fitted to the existing anatomy. Whether better long-term clinical results than with prosthesis designs of earlier generations are linked to these implants remains to be seen. Shoulder endoprostheses find clinical application in all forms of primary and secondary shoulder arthrosis, rheumatoid arthritis, humeral head necrosis, and non-reconstructable humeral head fractures.

Individual adaptation to the given anatomy of the prosthesis being implanted is possible

Indications:
shoulder arthrosis,
rheumatoid arthritis,
humeral head necrosis,
humeral head fractures

Consideration of various anatomical parameters is necessary

Shape, material, and fixation principles. To attain an anatomical reconstruction of the shoulder joint various anatomical parameters concerning prosthesis design as well as the later implantation by the surgeon must be taken into consideration.

Ante-/retroversion. The retroversion of the humeral joint surface to the transepicondylar axis of the elbow is not only interindividual, but also different between the right and left shoulders of the same person and falls somewhere between 0° und 55°.

Retroversion inter- und intraindividually different

Inclination. Through retroversion and the inclination angle – the angle between the anatomical neck and the metaphyseal stem axis – the resection level for the shoulder prosthesis implantation can be determined. The inclination angle falls on average between 30° and 55°.

Fixing of the resection level by retroversion and inclination angle

Offset. Offset is defined as the position of the centre of the humeral head in relation to the middle of the humeral stem. On average the centre of the humeral head is displaced around 0.004–0.14 m medially and 0.002–0.10 m posteriorly.

Offset: position of the center of the humeral head to the middle of the humeral stem

Various biomaterials can be applied in the production of shoulder endoprostheses. The materials used should show physical properties that are as similar as possible to the bone they are replacing. The most balanced relationship possible between stability and flexibility is important in order to prevent stress shielding.

Use of various biomaterials

Furthermore, the biological compatibility and resistance against wear and corrosion must be guaranteed. Materials frequently used are stainless steel, cobalt-chrome inserts and titanium for the prosthesis stems. For the glenoid component the synthetic polyethylene is usually used so that a metal/polyethylene joint combination comes about.

Stems made of stainless steel, cobalt-chrome alloys, titanium

Glenoid component made of polyethylene

The shoulder prostheses currently used usually offer the possibility of cemented as well as cementless application (Fig. 1.8). In this way the prosthesis is anchored mainly in the proximal humerus. In younger patients with bones of good quality cementless prostheses are preferably used, while in older patients with osteoporotic bones there is a tendency toward cemented implantation. A general guideline based on scientific data relating to this does not however currently exist.

Cemented and cement-free anchoring is possible

With younger patients preferably cementless, with older patients preferably cemented implantation

Modern cementing techniques with cement restrictors and retrograde cement insertion under pressure with a spray system and prior vacuum mixing are usually applied. Possible disadvantages of the use of bone cement are heat generation, heterogeneity of the cement layer, and the decreased solidity of the cement. Regarding materials, as well as rustproof cobalt-chrome inlays, stems made of titanium are used.

Use of bone cement

A cementless press-fit implantation of the shoulder prostheses has principle advantages with the same stability. These are effective particularly in younger, active patients, as reverse surgery on

Cement-free Press-fit implantation

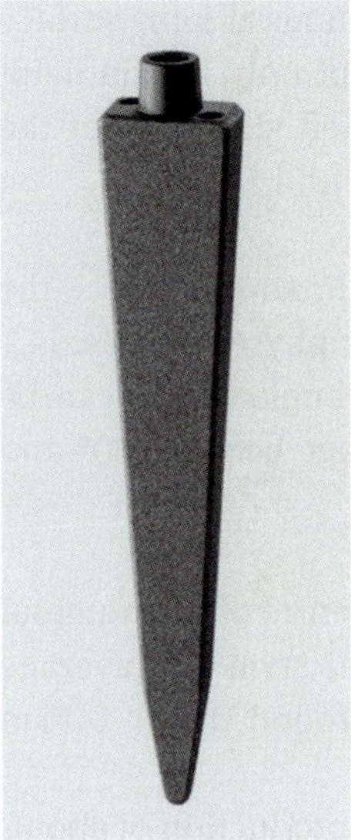

Fig. 1.8: Cement-free stem of the modular Promos prosthesis (Smith & Nephew).

the basis of young age is conceivable. The reversal of a cemented shoulder prosthesis is a technically demanding operation in which the humerus must usually be osteotomized in order to remove the prosthesis and the bone cement. In turn, this makes it hard to fix the revised stem.

Requirements of cementless implantation

With a cementless implant a corresponding primary stability must be guaranteed, in order to achieve safer ingrowth of the prosthesis. This must on the one hand be supported by the shape of the implant and on the other hand by a corresponding surface treatment. Thus, the basis of this rotational stability is already laid in the preparation of the medullary space, which is carried out with cutting of the medullary space specially adjusted to the prosthesis (Fig. 1.9).

The crafting of the surfaces of the implants is another important requirement for primary press-fit fixation. A rough structuring of the whole stem surface does lead to firm osseointegration; however, explantation of the stem in revision surgery is almost as difficult as with cemented implants. Modern shoulder prostheses, therefore, sit on a finely structured surface or on a purely proximal structuring of the fixation in order to minimize the distal application of force. For the treatment of the stem surface the possibility exists of raw radiation of the stem material (e.g. titanium) in the area of the stem, in which osteointegration is desired.

Structured surface or purely proximal structuring

Other methods of enlarging the contact surface between the prosthesis and bone

A special form of the structured surface is the so-called trabecular metal™, a material consisting of tantalum or carbon with a porous structure similar to bone. Another possibility for increasing the contact surface between the prosthesis and bone is coating the

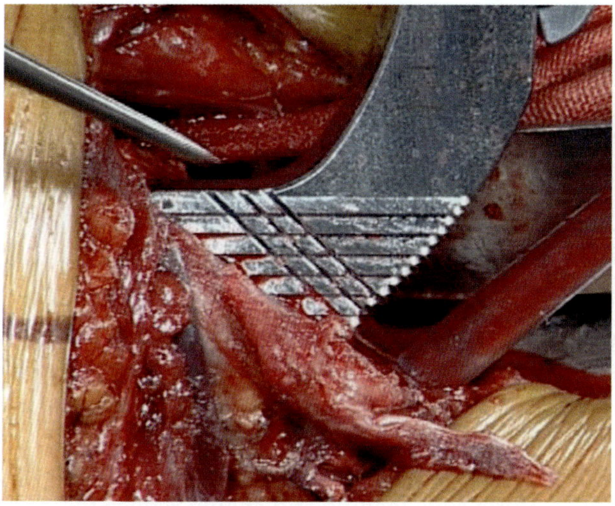

Fig. 1.9: Medullary cavity drill for the Promos prosthesis (Smith & Nephew).

prosthesis with hydroxyapatite, which has osteoconductive and osteointegrative effects.

1.4.2 Glenoid Replacement

The Neer mark I prosthesis was soon developed as a hemiprosthesis without glenoid replacement. Poor results on the basis of untreated glenoid arthrosis, however, led with the Neer mark II prosthesis to the possibility of replacing the glenoid increasing too. While complications in the area of the stem in the shoulder prosthesis are rare the glenoid component is seen as the critical part of the total shoulder endoprosthetic. Glenoid loosening is in up to 12.5 % the most frequent reason for revision surgery in total shoulder prosthesis.

Glenoid loosening of approximately 12.5 % is the most frequent cause of revision

For this reason numerous modifications of the original Neer glenoid replacement have been developed. Thus, the shape, the compliance with the ball, the fixation methods, and the material were changed in all kinds of variations. This multitude of variations proves that the ideal glenoid replacement has not yet been found.

Development of numerous modifications of the original Neer glenoid replacement

Shape, material, and fixation principles. The rear surface of the glenoid component is a basic shaped component. Here, convex and flat rear surfaces differ (Fig. 1.10a, b). The convex rear surface is the "anatomical" variant, as it takes into consideration the original anatomy of the glenoid. A potential advantage of a convex glenoid

Back surface of the glenoid component important shape component

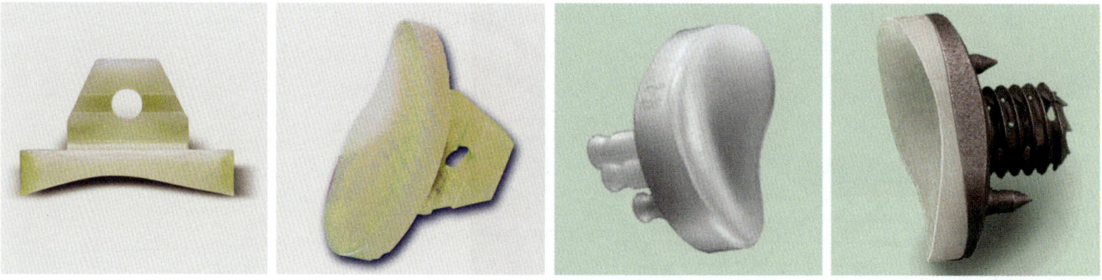

(a) (b) (c) (d)

Fig. 1.10: Cemented polyethylene glenoid with "Keel" and more planar (a) and convex (b) rear surface (Tornier). (c) Cemented "pegged" glenoid of the Promos prosthesis (Smith & Nephew). (d) Metal-backed glenoid with screw of the Univers prosthesis (Arthrex).

Differentiation between convex and flat back surfaces

component is the larger contact surface, which leads to equal distribution of the eccentric edge loading and should reduce the danger of loosening. A flat (non-compliant) glenoid component offers the theoretical advantage in the case of eccentric glenoid function of only having to adapt to the superior socket edge. Independently of the shape of the rear surface, the greatest congruence possible between the socket bearing and the glenoid component is required in order to reduce the risk of loosening.

Relationship between the humeral head radius and the glenoid radius = mismatch

Mismatch vital for implantation of a total shoulder prosthesis

The relationship between the radius of the humeral head and that of the glenoid, the so-called "mismatch" is decidedly significant for the implantation of a total shoulder prosthesis. A completely compliant humeral head–glenoid pairing leads to exact centralization of the humeral head and to the suppression of the physiological translation by so-called "concavity compression". This does not correspond to the anatomical relationship – a translation movement of 0.0015–0.002 m is regarded as being physiological. If the translation is forced by terminal movements, it amounts to peak loads at the border areas of the glenoid component. Early unilateral polyethylene use and loosening of the glenoid component by unilateral loading and the corresponding lifting load of the opposite side to that on which the loosening starts can occur. Matsem described this process as the "rocking horse phenomenon". A non-compliant humeral head–glenoid pairing with a larger glenoid radius is aimed for because it enables a more physiological translation of the component and concentrates the mechanical load in the more stable center of the glenoid. A so-called mismatch of the glenoid and radial head of 0.005–0.007 m in favor of the glenoid is considered an ideal compromise between the stability and translation of the total endoprosthesis.

Rocking horse phenomenon: glenoid loosening through asymmetrical load

The possibilities of secure fixation of the glenoid component are considerably hindered by the anatomical conditions of the glenoid, in particular in the case of advanced shoulder arthrosis, in comparison to other joints. In a normal glenoid the width of the spongy bone amounts to approximately 0.026 m and can in the case of advanced arthrosis decrease to 0.010–0.015 m or less. The aim with the design of a glenoid component is therefore to have to resect as little as possible of the already sparse existing bone, but still guarantee secure fixation. Cemented systems are currently in the majority.

Secure fixation of the glenoid component impeded considerably by the anatomy of the glenoid

Cemented glenoid components usually consist entirely of polyethylene. Here, too, two large groups differ from one another. A distinguishing feature is the shape of the prominent part of the rear surface through a central "keel" (Fig. 1.10a, b) or as several bolts, or "pegs" (Fig. 1.10c). Today, a centrally positioned keel, as originally developed by Charles Neer, is the design type most frequently used. A further development in the keel glenoid is that the keel is moved anteriorly in order to position the fixation more directly under the main starting point of the load onto the glenohumeral joint. Furthermore, the more compact posterior bone stock of the glenoid can still be preserved with this anterior fixation, while the weaker anterior part is resected within the implantation.

Predominantly cemented system

Two groups of cemented glenoid components: difference in the shape

of the prominent part of the back surface

- Most frequent design type: centrally positioned keel
- Fixation by bolts or spigots/valve = pegs

The use of several bolts or pegs as fixation offers the advantage of low usage of bone in the preparation of the socket bearing. Provided there is adequate space between the pegs, shear forces are thus also diminished in comparison to a central fixation with a comparatively large keel. The critical point in the use of the peg glenoid is the preparation, i.e., drilling holes for the pegs. With the multiplicity of holes there is a danger of the low bone stock of the glenoid weakening in several places and in extreme cases leading to fracture of the glenoid. Whether peg or keel fixation has a better prognosis with regard to the complication of socket loosening cannot be answered with certainty because of divergent study results. It is advisable to adapt to the anatomical features. This shows an advantage of the peg glenoid, i.e., adequate bone stock, at least experimentally. On the other hand, the keel glenoid seems to be able to guarantee better fixation if there is already marked erosion with considerable thinning of the glenoid.

Advantage of peg or keel fixation dependent on anatomical conditions

The approach to implanting a cementless glenoid is accompanied by a change in the material. Only with rear surfaces made of metal, the so-called metal-backed component, is there the possibility of actual biological ingrowth of the glenoid component into the existing bone. The primary fixation is carried out with, for example, screws. The metal-backed glenoid components usually consist of two components, the "metal back" itself and a polyethylene part, which articulates with the humeral head component (Fig. 1.10d).

Biological ingrowth of the glenoid component into

Existing bone only with rear surfaces {backs} made of metal (metal-backed)

Possible complications with the contact surface between two different materials

Thus, another contact surface is formed between two different materials, with possible complications, e.g., separation of the two parts or abrasion of the components. Other potential disadvantages of this glenoid are the increased width of the two components and/or the thinner polyethylene part and possible stress shielding of the underlying bone by the prime stable fixation.

1.4.3 Resurfacing

Reproduction of the normal anatomy with minimal bone resection

The concept of endoprosthetic resurfacing at the shoulder joint differs in various aspects from that of the conventional stem prosthesis. It is primarily based on the exclusive replacement of the destroyed joint surface with the reproduction of the normal anatomy using minimal bone resection.

Advantages of surface area replacement (cap prosthesis)

Particularly in young patients with good bone quality this so-called cap prosthesis offers the possibility of replacing the diseased cartilage surface without having to handle the humeral stem. In the case of reverse surgery this makes it easier for the surgeon to anchor the revision stem because, even with the explantation of the cap prosthesis, the stem does not have to be handled.

Disadvantage: by impeded exposure of the glenoid, more difficult glenoid replacement

In 2006: approximately 1,500 cap prostheses/10,000 implanted shoulder prostheses

A potential technical disadvantage of all cap prosthesis surgery results from the distinctly impeded exposure of the glenoid. Glenoid replacement is thus considerably more difficult. In advanced arthrosis or necrosis with glenoid involvement this disadvantage should be considered and the indication for resurfacing critically reviewed. The increasing popularity of such systems emphasizes the fact that in Germany in 2006, out of approximately 10,000 implanted shoulder prostheses, approximately 1,500 resurfacing implants were implanted.

Cemented and cementless resurfacing implants

Various resurfacing designs

Shape, material, and fixation principles. Even with resurfacing there is a choice of cemented as well as cementless implants. The Scan Cup is a hemispherical cap made of stainless steel measuring initially 0.003 m and later 0.0017 m thick (Fig. 1.11). Channels running around the inside of the cap, as well as radially, secure the fixation of the prosthesis and allow expulsion of the excess cement. The edge of the prosthesis tapers in cross-section. Another example of cemented resurfacing is the Durom™ shoulder cup developed by Rüther in 1996 (Fig. 1.12). This cemented resurfacing prosthesis is currently available in seven different sizes (0.040–0.052 m). The inside of the cap is coarsely finished for better binding with the bone cement. Because of a centrally positioned cylindrical peg the prosthesis is centered when struck and the cap on the spherically milled humeral head is prevented from tilting.

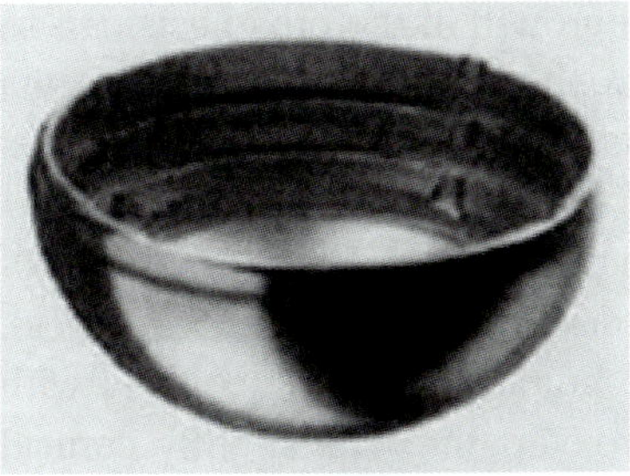

Fig. 1.11: Scan Shoulder®
(MITAB, Sjöbo, Sweden).

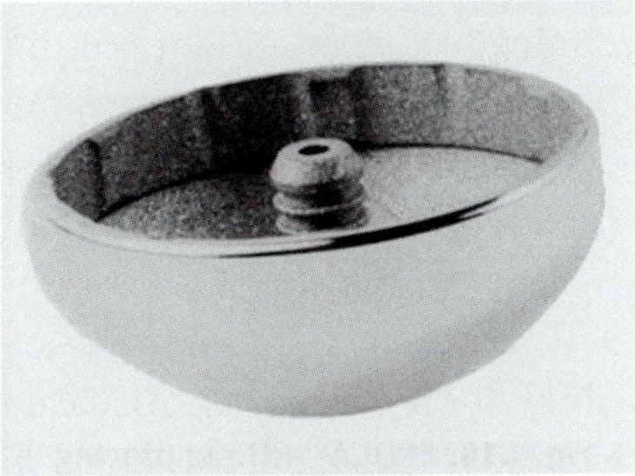

Fig. 1.12: Durom™ Shoulder Cup
(Zimmer, Germany).

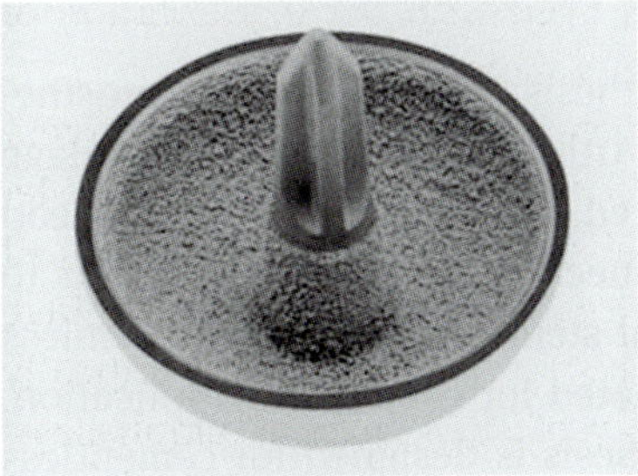

Fig. 1.13: Global C.A.P.™
(Depuy, Kirkel Limbach, Germany).

Longest clinical experience with the Copeland™ cup

After the Scan Cup, the Copeland™ Shoulder is the resurfacing implant with the longest clinical experience. This cementless implant is currently available in eight different sizes. The radius of curvature measures 0.050 or 0.054 m. However, with differing ball sizes varying anatomical measurements and offsets are covered.

Structure of the Copeland™ cup

The cup itself is manufactured from a cobalt-chrome-molybdenum alloy and features an interior coated with hydroxyapatite, as well as improved ingrowth characteristics. The conically shaped press-fit peg supplied with anchoring ridges should guarantee rotational stability (Fig. 1.4).

Conceptional features of Global-C.A.P.™ resurfacing

The Global C.A.P.™ resurfacing prosthesis by Dupuy (Fig. 1.13) displays similar conceptional features to the Copeland prosthesis. This is also a cementless implant. The osteointegration was supported by a so-called Porocoat® coating on the underside of the prosthesis. Characteristic of this coating are randomly distributed beads with appropriate pore size. With an additional hydroxyapatite coating (Duo-Fix™) the bone ingrowth of the prosthesis can be further accelerated. In contrast to the Copeland prosthesis, the press-fit peg, which is also equipped with fixation ridges, is cross-shaped and tapers at the front.

Fixation principle f the EPOCA®-RH resurfacing prosthesis

A completely different fixation principle is shown by the EPOCAE®-RH resurfacing prosthesis, developed by Hertel (Synthes). The epiphyseal fixation within the humeral head is achieved with a perforated cap coated with hydroxyapatite. The slightly conical shape of the cap enables good primary press-fit stability (Fig. 1.14).

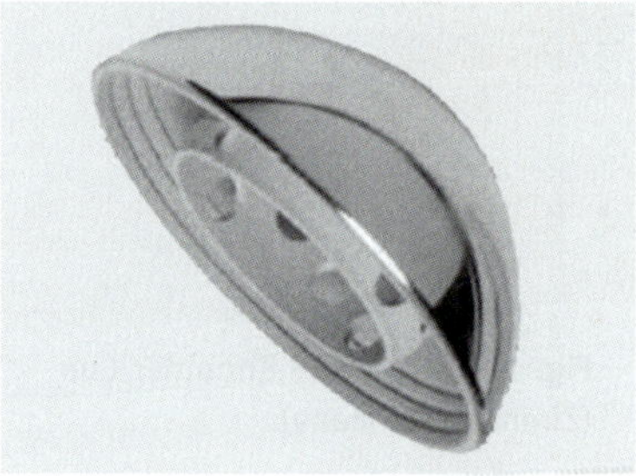

Fig. 1.14: EPOCA®-RH resurfacing prosthesis (Synthes, Schweiz).

Design and fixation of the stemless humeral head prosthesis “Eclipse”

In contrast to the classic cap prosthesis, with the Eclipse prosthesis, developed by Habermayer for Arthrex, not only is the cartilage up to the subchondral bone removed, but the whole humeral head is resected along the anatomical neck of the humerus similar to the implantation of a conventional stem prosthesis. This stemless humeral head prosthesis is designated for cementless application. This stemless humeral head prosthesis is designed for cementless application and consists of a ball (cobalt-chrome-molybdenum alloy), a pressure disk and a screw (both titanium alloy; Fig. 1.15). The ball is placed over a cone-shaped socket onto the pressure disk, which is available in different diameters. With a total of six ridges on the bone contact side stable fixation of the pressure disk is enabled. The fixation in the humerus is eventually done using

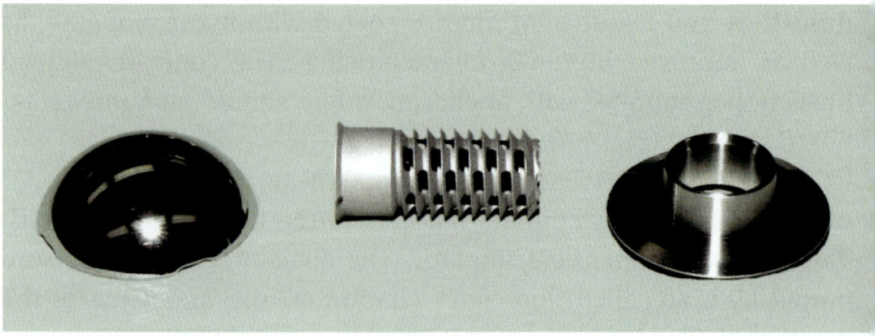

Fig. 1.15: Eclipse™ humeral head prosthesis (Arthrex, Karlsfeld, Deutschland).

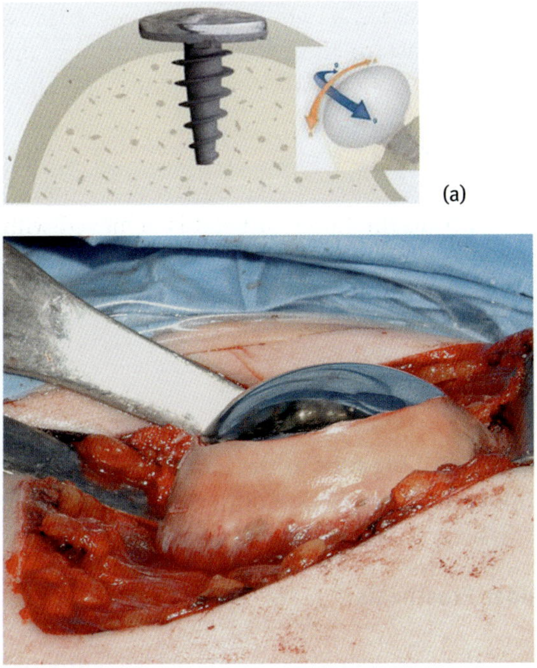

(a)

(b)

Fig. 1.16: (a, b) HemiCAP resurfacing (Arthrosurface Inc., Franklin, Massachusetts, USA).

the screw. Slits along the thread of the screw allow the ingrowth of spongy bone and in addition lead to a corundum-blasted surface to lasting osseointegration and secure fixation. With this prosthesis, the implantation of a glenoid component is not impeded by "normal" resection of the humeral head.

Individual reconstruction of smaller cartilage injuries of the humeral head with HemiCAP® resurfacing

An even more individual reconstruction, in particular of smaller cartilage injuries of the humeral head, is permitted by the so-called HemiCAP® resurfacing prosthesis (Arthrosurface Inc., Franklin, Massachusetts, USA; Fig. 1.16). This consists of two parts: a graphite screw made of titanium for implant fixation as well as an articulation surface made of cobalt-chrome, which is available in three different sizes (0.025 m, 0.030 m, 0.035 m). Various offset sizes correspond to the superior–inferior as well as to the mediolateral curve radius on the implantation side. As a result, intraoperatively, an exact reproduction of the original anatomical joint surface is possible.

Arthrex also offers resurfacing for the proximal humerus with the "Partial Eclipse" (Fig. 1.17). This is additionally characterized by the ability to be implanted arthroscopically and thus without removal of the subscapularis tendon. All instruments and implant components are introduced via ventral access into the joint in the

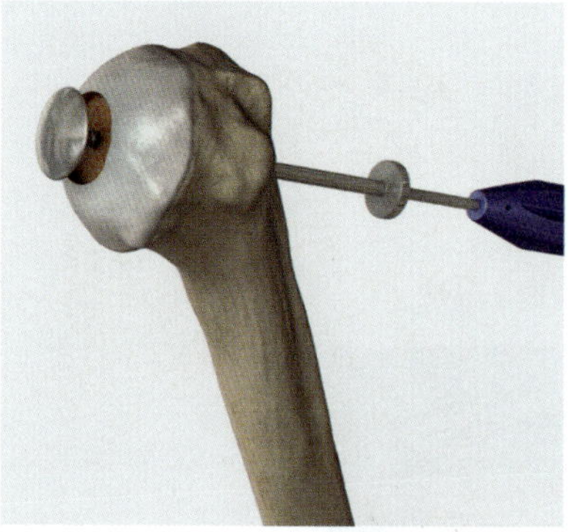

Fig. 1.17: Partial Eclipse resurfacing (Arthrex).

rotator cuff interval and a drilling tube at the humeral head. However, at the moment, long-term results are not yet available.

1.4.4 Reverse Shoulder Prosthesis

Biomechanical principle of reverse prosthesis: reversal of the anatomical relationship between glenoid and humeral components

- Prototype: Delta III prosthesis
- Prevention of early loosening
- Disadvantage: no reproduction of rotation
- Indication: defect arthropathy

A particular problem of the shoulder endoprosthesis is confronted when shoulder arthrosis involves an extensive rotator cuff rupture. This so-called defect arthropathy represents a special case and requires a specific solution in order to enable secure implantation with functional improvement of the shoulder function. The aim of reproducing the original anatomy cannot be achieved in this situation; it requires a complete change in the joint biomechanics. The biomechanical principle of the reverse prosthesis affects the reversal of the anatomical relationship between the glenoid and humeral components. The prototype of the modern reverse prosthesis is the Delta III prosthesis, developed by Paul Grammont, which achieves sufficient mobility around a stable center of rotation by medialization and distalization in this difficult biomechanical situation (Fig. 1.18). Thus, the lever of the deltoid muscle is lengthened. The glenoid component was therefore larger than in earlier prosthesis designs and the humeral application was oriented almost horizontally at 155°. By articulating the convex glenoid body with a concave joint partner in the humerus, a stable center of rotation for the whole range of movement is reproduced. With this modification of the prosthesis designs, the problem of early loosening is resolved. A known functional limitation of the reverse prosthesis is that rotation, external rotation in particular, in contrast to flexion and abduction, cannot be reproduced.

The primary indication for reverse shoulder prosthesis is defect arthropathy. For this indication the most long-term and best results are to be found in the literature. Recently, however, the reverse

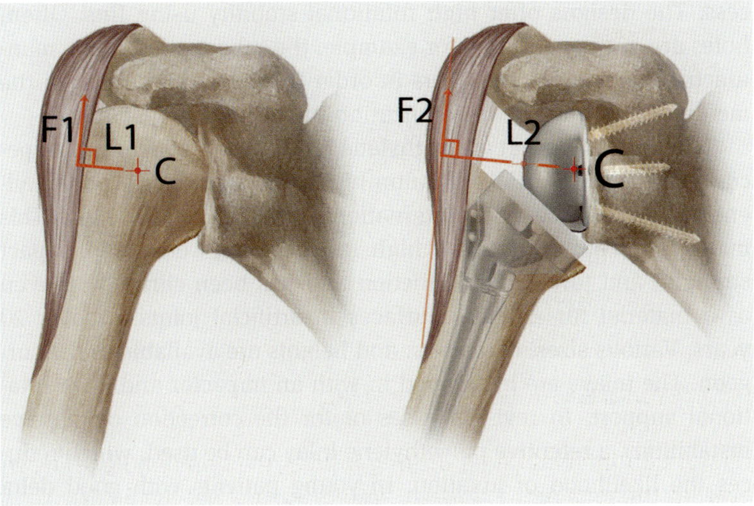

Fig. 1.18: (a, b) Basic principle of the reverse prosthesis: 1. Fixed and medialized center of rotation (extension of the lever arm of the Delta (L2 > L1) and decrease in the torque on the glenoid components, and 2. Enlargement of the acromiohumeral gap for reconstruction of the Delta's tension (F2 > F1) (De Puy).

prosthesis has become increasingly used as a revision implant and in unreconstructable fractures in older patients. In spite of the encouraging results there is a high complication rate; thus, the indication should be evaluated critically. Use in younger patients is generally not recommended.

- Mostly used as a revision implant
- High complication rate

Shape, Material, and Fixation Principles. With the modular system of modern prosthesis systems it is possible to customize the prosthesis. For this purpose stems of various lengths and diameters, different metaphyses, polyethylene inlays of different heights and diameters (which could also be extended with adapters) and glenopsheres with diameters suitable for methaphyses are supplied (Fig. 1.6). The stems are usually made of cobalt-chrome, they are polished at the distal end, and adapted to the stem anatomy using cone geometry. Some manufacturers coat the stems at the proximal end with porous Ti_6Al_4V. This alloy possesses high mechanical strength properties, permits osteointegration through direct adhesion of the bone to the roughened surfaces, and offers low resistance to wear. The length of the coated part varies among different manufacturers. The stems are available in various lengths and diameters and can be inserted with or without cement. The epiphysis usually consists of the same material and is fixed to the stem using various screwing systems. Like the technique for the stem, an epiphysis must be chosen for the cemented or cementless pro-

Individual prosthesis adaptation through modular systems

- Stems with various lengths, diameters, coatings, various metaphyses cess. The designs offer high rotational stability using fins. Often, holes are put in to attach, for example, the tuberosities. Some manufacturers carry place holders in order to bridge the defects in the metaphysis or increase lateralization in the case of instability.

▸ Humeral insert (polyethylene inlay) in various heights and diameters

The humeral insert (polyethylene inlay) consists mainly of a special polyethylene UHMWPE (ultra-high-molecular-weight polyethylene in accordance with International Standard ISO5834-2). This material is characterized by high resistance to wear, high impact strength, and low dynamic friction and has been clinically proven as a material for articular surfaces in artificial joints for over 20 years. Various sizes, diameters, and heights are available to the surgeon. The inlays are hammered in with an impactor and have rotational support. In revision cases or for the correction of massive instabilities, a retentive polyethylene inlay can be used, which reduces the likelihood of luxation. In young patients with good delta voltage a high-mobility inlay can be deployed if necessary. This features little concavity and thus permits a greater range of motion.

▸ Glenospheres with diameters to fit metaphyses

The glenosphere usually consists of a CoCrMo forge alloy in accordance with ISO5832-12, a known and approved material with great wear resistance in materials testing. They are available with various diameters, from most manufacturers at 0.036 and 0.042 m. The glenosphere is mostly pressed onto the glenoid base with an impactor, and then secured with a central blocking screw.

Glenoids are mostly plates fixed without cement

The glenoids (metaglenoid and metaglene) are usually plates that can be fixed without cement, for which the various manufacturers provide very different concepts. The sizes vary from manufacturer to manufacturer and are non-compliant so that the right head size has to be found. With most manufacturers the fixation of the base plate is achieved without cement through a central peg and two to four peripheral, mostly fixed-angle screws (Fig. 1.19).

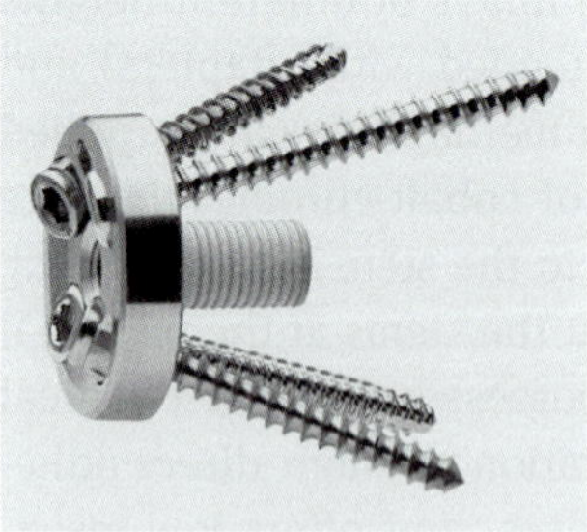

Fig. 1.19: Glenospheres of the Aequalis Reversed prosthesis with two cortical screws (anterior and posterior) (Tornier).

1.4.5 Perspective

The most recent stage of development comprises the fifth generation modular prostheses, which, if required, enable the transformation of a conventional shoulder prosthesis with or without a stem and glenoid into an reverse shoulder prosthesis. If there is advanced degeneration of the rotator cuff, such revision surgery can be facilitated considerably as the stem as well as the glenoid plate can be retained. For example, the Promos shoulder system by Smith & Nephew offers the possibility of attaching a humeral cup to a conventional stem and, after implantation of the reverse cementless glenoid component, converting a hemiprosthesis into a reverse prosthesis without explanting the original stem (Fig. 1.7). In addition, partial resurfacing, if there is a strong indication, is a good innovation and alternative in shoulder endoprosthetics. In particular, the arthroscopically implantable brands are interesting with regard to protecting soft tissue and have the potential for good long-term results. However, this remains to be seen.

Fifth-generation modular prostheses the current state of development

Transformation of a conventional shoulder prosthesis with or without a stem and glenoid into a reverse shoulder prosthesis is possible

Partial resurfacing is a good alternative if there is a strong indication

1.5 Indications and Contraindications

Persistent and progressive shoulder pain requiring medication as well as increasing limitation of movement owing to stiffening of the shoulder in radiologically verified arthrotic changes are indications for shoulder prosthesis implantation. The characteristics of radiological parameters, such as the size of the joint space and socket morphology, are thus secondary to the presenting pathology.

Indications for shoulder prosthesis implantation based on symptoms

Typical indications for a shoulder endoprosthesis are:

- Primary shoulder arthrosis
- Post-traumatic shoulder arthrosis
- Avascular humeral head necrosis
- Rheumatoid arthritis
- Instability arthrosis
- Defect arthropathy

Typical indications

1.5.1 Primary Shoulder Arthrosis

In comparison to the statically loaded joints of the lower extremities, primary shoulder arthrosis is diagnosed less frequently and has a comparatively low prevalence of about 3 %. However, it should by no means be overlooked in the diagnostics of shoulder pain. The pain symptoms mostly begin diffusely and only seldom suggest the glenohumeral joint as being the primary cause of pain. Patients complain about pain at rest or with motion, but this mostly does not lead to any functionally relevant limitation of shoulder movement. Not until the advanced stage does it corre-

Primary shoulder arthrosis

- ▸ Prevalence approximately 3 %
- ▸ Symptoms

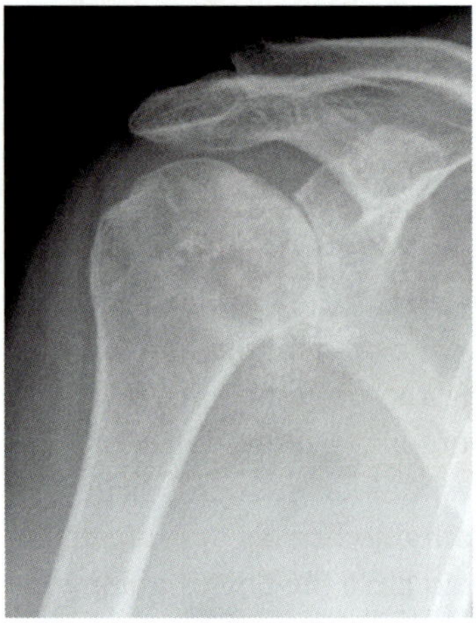

Fig. 1.20: Primary shoulder arthrosis on non-contrast radiography.

spond to increasing limitation of movement in which rotational movements in particular are considerably reduced. Radiologically, narrowing of the joint space does not make any clear appearance in the early stages.

▸ Radiological signs of arthrosis at the progressive stage

In the advanced stage the typical radiological signs of arthrosis are found, such as subchondral sclerosis of the joint surfaces, the formation of humeral collar osteophytes and subchondral ganglionic cysts, right up to the complete deformation of the humeral head (Fig. 1.20). As a further, typically pathomorphological correlate, shrinking of the frontal as well as enlargement of the lower articular capsule are found. The rotator cuff is mostly intact in primary shoulder arthrosis. In the case of a central humeral head position with physiological concavity of the joint socket only a humeral head replacement in the form of a hemiprosthesis is possible. In all other cases, in particular if there is dorsal glenoid wastage, a total endoprosthesis should be preferred for primary shoulder arthrosis, because the risk of the loosening of an artificial glenoid replacement is significantly combated.

▸ Rotator cuff mostly intact

▸ Hemiprosthesis or (mostly) total endoprosthesis

1.5.2 Humeral Head Necrosis

Humeral head necrosis

▸ Post-traumatic or non-traumatic form

Humeral head necrosis usually forms the basis of a circulatory disorder of multifactorial genesis. At the same time, it is necessary to differentiate between a post-traumatic form as a consequence of a humeral head fracture and a non-traumatic form. The latter most frequently occurs after local or systemic cortisone therapy. Other frequent causes are alcohol abuse, Cushing syndrome, hemoglo-

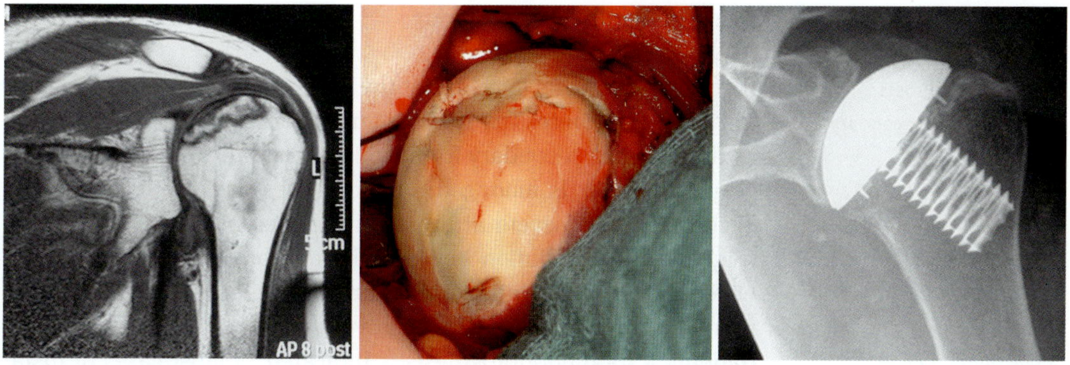

(a) (b) (c)

Fig. 1.21: (a, b) Humeral head necrosis on MRT and intraoperatively after high-dose chemotherapy. (c) Postoperative X-ray after implantation of a stemless Eclipse prosthesis (Arthrex).

binopathies, Gaucher's disease, and pancreatitis (Fig. 1.21a, b). The increasing destruction of the humeral head and/or of the whole joint takes place according to Cruess' classification system of radiological criteria stages I–V. On the basis of the fact that in humeral head necrosis for a long time a considerable discrepancy between the very forceful destruction of the humeral head and the only slight change in the glenoid joint partner was apparent, there is in most cases no indication for socket replacement (Fig. 1.21c).

- Cause: circulatory disorder of multifactorial genesis
- Mostly no indication for socket replacement

1.5.3 Rheumatoid Arthritis

In rheumatoid arthritis the shoulder joint is not normally the primary affected joint. In addition to the pathognomonic inflammation of the synovial membrane, which leads to destruction of the joint surfaces of the humeral head and glenoid, it often results in premature injury to the rotator cuff. Second, it can result in humeral head elevation, depending on the extent of the rotator cuff injury. Indication and implant choice in rheumatoid arthritis are largely determined by the degree of joint surface destruction (humeral and especially glenoidal) and the state of the rotator cuff. With sufficient glenoid bone substance and intact rotator cuff the implantation of a total shoulder endoprosthesis can by all means be contemplated. If there is more advanced glenoid destruction and/or an existing rotator cuff defect, the use of a shoulder hemiprosthesis is indicated. If there is sufficient bony substance of the humeral head and/or just in younger patients, resurfacing can be considered, as an alternative to the conventional stem prosthesis.

Rheumatoid arthritis

- Often premature damage to the rotator cuff
- Indication and choice of implant depend on the degree of destruction of the joint surface and condition of the rotator cuff

1.5.4 Instability Arthrosis

Instability arthrosis
- Primary and secondary form

Instability arthrosis develops at the base of one or several shoulder luxations. It is necessary to distinguish between primary instability arthrosis and a secondary form, which arises after stabilization surgery. The latter is among the main causes in 55-year-olds of the occurrence of a severe arthrosis in the area of the shoulder joint (Fig. 1.22). A correlation between the number of luxations experienced and the forming of the arthrosis does not exist for the primary form. In spite of the relatively young average age of the patients a total endoprosthesis is indicated in most cases of instability arthrosis, because the socket is mostly arthrotically changed and dorsal subluxation persists. The original problem was indeed an instability problem that indicated the necessity of good concavity of the socket. Second, especially posteriorly, there is danger of erosion of the socket, which would lead to recurrent instability if a socket replacement were lacking. In the special case of a chronically stuck front or back luxation with corresponding destruction of the edge of the sockets and humeral head compression fracture a hemiprosthesis is indicated. In some cases the socket damage should be balanced by appropriate surface milling in order to prevent recurrent luxation. Only in certain cases is bone socket construction necessary.

- Mostly total endoprosthesis indicated

Indication for a hemiprosthesis in special cases

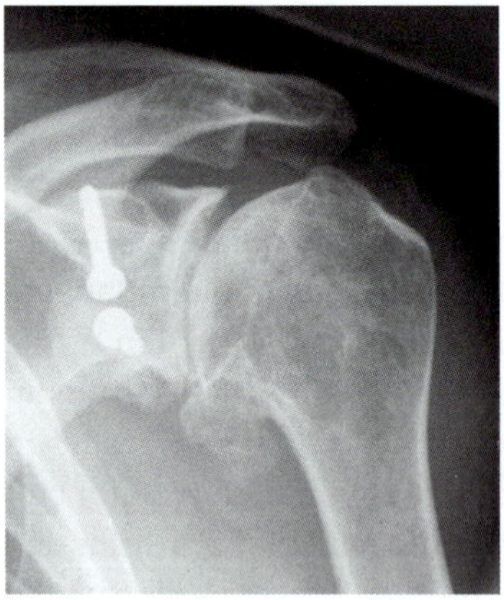

Fig. 1.22: Secondary instability arthrosis on non-contrast radiography.

1.5.5 Post-traumatic Shoulder Arthrosis

Post-traumatic omarthrosis

Post-traumatic arthrosis arises after conservative or surgical treatment of humeral head fractures (Fig. 1.23). They mostly represent complex situations as a combination of bone defects and injuries

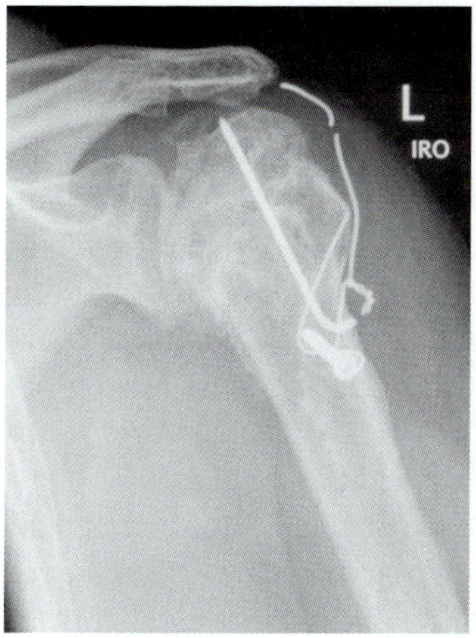

Fig. 1.23: Post-traumatic shoulder arthrosis on non-contrast radiography.

of the rotator cuff and pectoral girdle musculature exists. As with instability arthrosis, glenoid arthrosis often exists, even in the post-traumatic situation, so that, if technically feasible, the implantation of a glenoid replacement should be liberally taken into consideration. New stemless prosthesis types, e.g., the Eclipse prosthesis (Arthrex) may enable the simplification of endoprosthetics provision (Fig. 1.5).

- After conservative or surgical treatment of humeral head fractures
- Implantation of a glenoid replacement

1.5.6 Defect Arthropathy

The defect arthropathy is characterized by the simultaneous presence of joint destruction as defined by shoulder arthrosis and marked defect of the rotator cuff, which leads to elevation of the humeral head under the acromion and variably distinct instability (Fig. 1.24a, b). Neer described this clinical picture in 1981 as "cuff tear arthropathy". The endoprosthetic joint replacement in the case of a defect arthrography represents a particular challenge owing to the rotator cuff defect. While conventional glenoid replacement in defect arthropathy is obsolete owing to premature loosening by the eccentric load ("rocking horse phenomenon"), a conventional shoulder hemiprosthesis often yields unsatisfactory results. To compensate for instability and loss of function, implantation of a reverse shoulder prosthesis is offered to patients over 70 years of age with a defect arthropathy (Fig. 1.24c).

Defect arthropathy
- Simultaneous presence of a shoulder arthrosis and rotator cuff defect

- Implantation of an reverse shoulder prosthesis

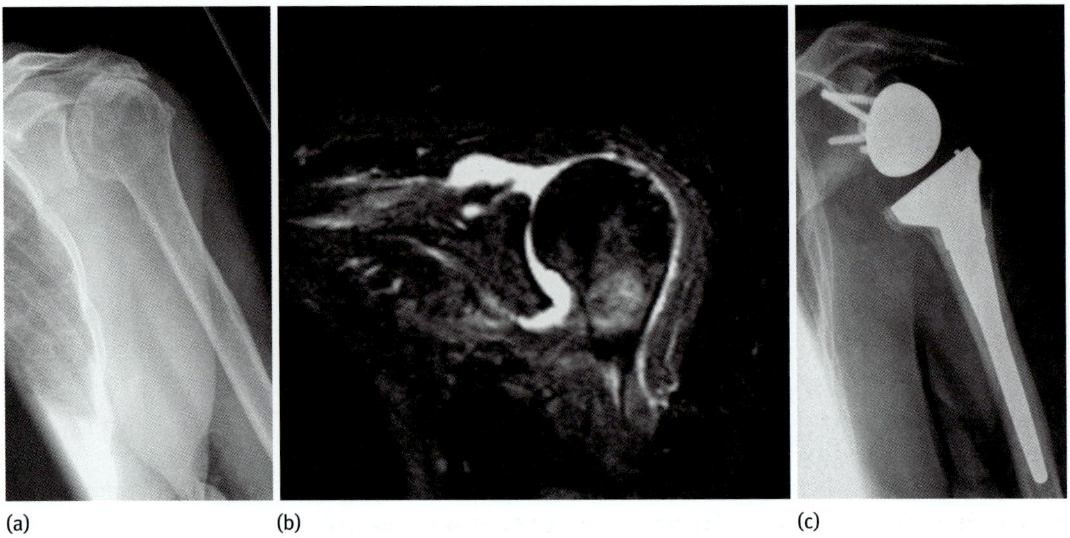

Fig. 1.24: (a, b) Defect arthropathy on non-contrast radiography and on MRT. (c) Postoperatively after reverse shoulder prosthesis.

1.5.7 Contraindications

Contraindications

Contraindications include:
- Florid local or systemic infections
- Inadequate bone socket to support the components in the proximal humerus or in the glenoid cavity
- Bad bone quality, e.g., in osteoporosis, which can result in considerable migration of the prosthesis and/or the danger of a fracture of the humerus or glenoid
- Neurological diseases such as myopathies, neurogenic arthropathy
- Septic arthritis

1.6 Surgical Technique

1.6.1 Surgical Planning

Routine MRT for the evaluation of the osseous conditions at the glenoid and depiction of the rotator cuff

Among the preoperative diagnostics in the planning of a shoulder endoprosthesis is an instrumental diagnosis in the form of conventional radiography in true anteroposterior and axial projections. Furthermore, cross-sectional imaging is routinely carried out for secure evaluation of the osseous conditions at the glenoid, as well as depiction of the rotator cuff. Magnetic resonance tomography (MRT) usually allows accurate evaluation of the rotator cuff as well as osseous deformity of the humeral head and glenoid. If there is a special problem regarding osseous conditions, computed tomography with 3D reconstruction, if necessary, should additionally be carried out, as this permits the pathology to be depicted accurately.

CT if there are special problems

For preoperative choice of implant, X-ray templates from all prosthesis manufacturers are usually available, although the appropriate enlargement factors have to be taken into consideration.

X-ray templates for the preoperative choice of implant

1.6.2 Total Shoulder Endoprosthesis

Surgical technique

The intervention is typically carried out under endotracheal anesthesia and is combined with an interscalene catheter for peri- and postoperative pain therapy. The patient is typically seated in the beach chair position (Fig. 1.25) with the upper body raised to approximately 45°. It is vital to place the patient sideways on the operating table in order to enable the upper arm to be lowered and extended at the edge of the table.

- Seating of the patient in the beach chair position

The classical deltoideopectoral approach is used as standard access point. After searching for the cephalic vein in Mohrenheim's space, the preparation of the deltoideopectoral sulcus are carried out from proximal to distal. After application of the retractors, the so-called "conjoined tendons" (short head biceps muscle and coracobrachialis) as well as the subscapularis tendon are depicted. Special attention should be given to the course of the axillary nerve, which curves dorsally to the underside of the subscapularis muscle and traverses the lateral axillary space.

- Standard access of the classical deltoideopectoral approach

Dependent on the preoperative ability for external rotation, the removal of the subscapularis tendon is carried out (0.005–0.010 m)

- Removal of the subscapularis tendon

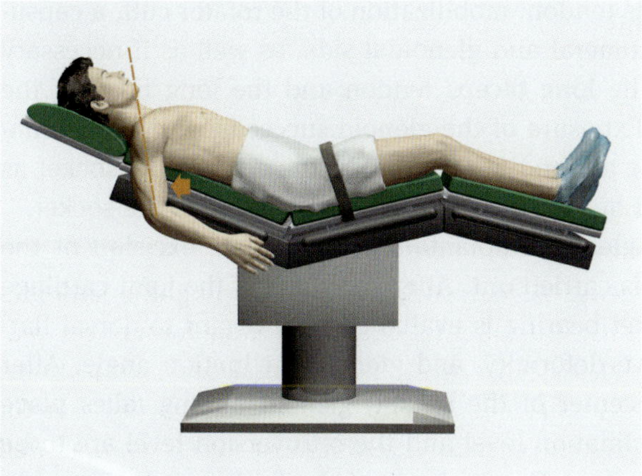

Fig. 1.25: Beach chair position.

medial of the approach to the lesser tuberosity (external rotation over 20°) or rather directly at the lesser tuberosity (external rotation 0–20°), as through the later additional medialization of the enthesis an additional increase in movement is possible. If there is severe contracture a complete subscapularis removal with bifocal capsulotomy is carried out.

▸ Luxation of the shoulder joint, humeral head resection, medullary cavity preparation

In addition, the shoulder joint luxation is successfully treated under careful external rotation, adduction, and extension. The typical humeral collar osteophytes are removed for exact representation of the resection level at the anatomical neck of the humerus. This is particularly important in order to avoid a size misidentification and the resultant overstuffing. A resection model can facilitate humeral head resection, which is performed with an inclination of approximately 125–140° and a retrotorsion of 20–30°. With the use of a conventional stem prosthesis, the medullary cavity preparation is done after the head resection.

Alternatively, however, a stemless prosthesis variant can be chosen for which preparation of the medullary cavity is omitted. After medullary cavity and/or ball preparation 4–5 transosseous sutures are presented for subscapularis tendon reattachment through the cortical neck of the humerus approximately 0.1 m below the resection surface. Through this medialization of the tendon, a gain of approximately 20° of external rotation is made.

▸ Subscapularis tendon reattachment

With the implantation of a total endoprosthesis the humeral head resection level is protected with an appropriate protective plate.

▸ Socket implantation

The technically most difficult surgical step is without doubt the socket implantation. A clear glenoid depiction of the glenoid, which is achieved through a complete release of soft tissue, is vital. A complete release soft tissue consists of the complete removal of the subscapularis tendon, mobilization of the rotator cuff, a capsulotomy on the humeral and glenoidal side, as well as if necessary a tenotomy of the long biceps tendon and the long head of the triceps muscle. Exposure of the glenoid succeeds with two Hohmann hooks at the top and at the front of the edge of the socket as well as a special head retractor over the rear edge of the socket.

▸ Complete release of soft tissue

In planned glenoid implantation a complete excision of the glenoid labrum is carried out. After curettage of the joint cartilage the cortical socket bearing is evaluated with regard to dorsal flattening, biconcave deformity, and glenoid inclination angle. After marking of the center of the socket, glenoid milling takes place in which the inclination level and the retroversion level are to be corrected if necessary. On the basis of the fairly soft bony conditions of the glenoid, the milling should be performed only just up to the subchondral bone. After milling the socket bearing has to be congruent with the glenoid component, because otherwise premature loosening of the socket is a danger.

In addition, the implanting of the definitive glenoid component is carried out (Fig. 1.26), where there must be differentiation between cemented and cementless glenoid replacements, so-called "metal-backs". After completion of the socket implantation, the implantation of the humeral head component is performed and the inspection of joint play, balancing, and stability (Fig. 1.27). The aim should be a dorsal head translation of 0.015 m as well as an abduction ability of at least 90°, internal rotational ability of 70°, and external rotational ability of 40°. After repositioning and definitive prosthesis implantation a careful readaptation of the subscapularis

- Implantation of the humeral head component
- Inspection of joint play, balancing, stability
- Concluding steps

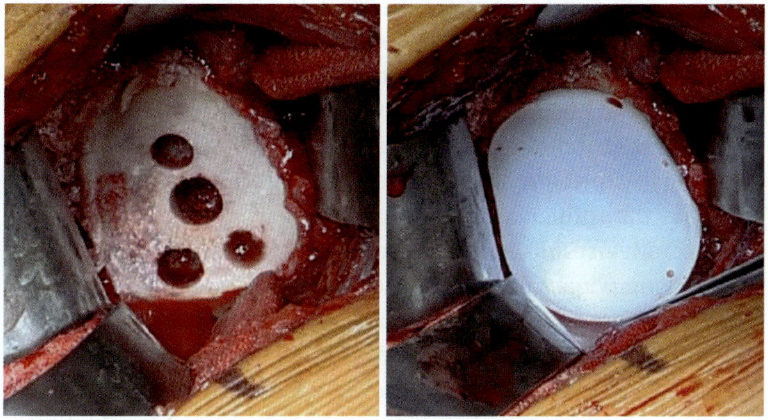

(a) (b)

Fig. 1.26: (a, b) Implantation of a cemented "pegged" glenoid.

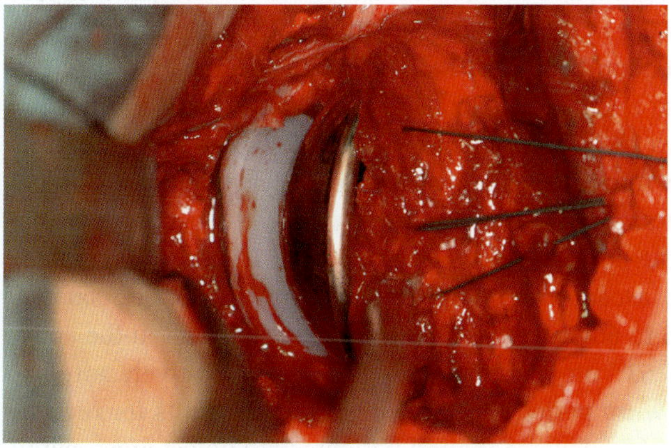

Fig. 1.27: Inspection of "joint play".

tendon in an easy abduction and external rotation position is essential. The sutures provided at the neck of the humerus are for reinsertion. To finish, the closing of the rotator cuff interval with a side-to-side suture of the subscapularis and supraspinatus takes place.

1.7 Results

Good results for pain reduction and functional improvement

In the course of the last decades the modern shoulder prosthesis has increasingly proved that, like hip and knee endoprosthetics, with the correct diagnosis reliably good results with regard to pain reduction and functional improvement are possible.

Total shoulder endoprosthesis: significantly better results in postoperative function, pain relief, mobilization than with the hemiprosthesis

Glenoid degeneration after hemisprosthesis

Glenoid component loosening after total endoprosthesis

The advantages of a shoulder hemiprosthesis are the technically less difficult intervention, less blood loss, shorter operating times, and lower costs. In a meta-analysis it could be shown that patients with a primary concentric shoulder arthrosis after implantation of a total shoulder prosthesis end up significantly better off with regard to postoperative function, pain relief, and movement. After shoulder hemiprosthesis 20 % of the patients had a secondary glenoid implantation. However, further long-term results are also necessary with the newer prosthesis models in order to be able to evaluate the influence of continual glenoid degeneration on the postoperative result after hemiprosthesis and/or loosening of the glenoid component after total endoprosthesis.

Advantages and disadvantages of resurfacing

So far, results for the resurfacing of the humeral head are available, in particular for rheumatoid arthritis and shoulder arthrosis. These correspond largely to the newer generation modular prostheses. The disadvantage of resurfacing is the extremely technically difficult implantation of a glenoid component. On the other hand a possible system change to a stem prosthesis is technically simple.

Best clinical results in primary shoulder arthrosis, worse in rheumatoid arthritis

The best clinical results using resurfacing were attained for patients with primary shoulder arthrosis. Copeland et al. achieved a constant score of 73.5 % after hemiprosthesis as well as 93.7 % after total endoprosthesis. Patients with rheumatoid arthritis showed worse results in the constant score than patients with primary shoulder arthrosis. In addition, in this patient cohort significantly higher rates of loosening of up to 25 % were found.

Defect arthropathy: best clinical results with reverse prosthesis

In patients with a defect arthropathy the reverse prosthesis has emerged as the implant with the best clinical results. Boileau et al. were able to ascertain an improvement in the average constant score from 18 to 66 points, as well as an improvement in the active flexion from 53° preoperatively to 123° postoperatively after an average follow-up period of 40 months.

Reverse prosthesis as a revision implant

As the results for revision implants are indeed worse than in patients with defect arthropathy, this difficult group of patients benefited significantly from the implantation of a reverse prosthesis. Boileau et al. observed a so-called "scapular notching", i.e., the cavity of the lower joint socket underneath the glenosphere.

Cavity of the lower joint socket below the glenoid sphere in 68 %

1.8 Complications

The total complication rate of shoulder endoprosthesis is stated in the literature as being 16 %. Within that we have to differentiate between intra- and postoperative as well as between general and prosthesis-specific complications.

Overall complication rate 16 %

Infections after shoulder prosthesis occur with a prevalence of 0.7 %. The most frequent pathogens are *Staphylococcus aureus*, *S. epidermidis*, and *Propionibacterium acnes*. The risk of an intraoperative periprosthetic fracture lies at around 1.1 %. Postoperative periprosthetic fractures show a frequency of 0.7 %. Neurological complications appear with a probability of under 1 %. In over 50 % of cases the axillary nerve is affected. In over two thirds of all neurological complications it corresponds to a Resitutio ad integrum. The prevalence of postoperative ruptures of the rotator cuff is 1.3 %, although in over half of all ruptures the subscapularis tendon is affected.

Prevalence of various complications

The risk of glenohumeral instabilities after shoulder prosthesis implantation is around 5 % and thereby represents the second overall most frequent complication. In over 80 % of cases it corresponds to superior or anterior instability whose cause is often multifactorial (neurogenic, muscular, capsular or implant-related).

Second most frequent complication: glenohumeral instabilities

Almost 40 % of all complications after shoulder endoprosthesis involve loosening of the prosthesis. Overall, the prevalence is 6.3 %. Over 80 % of all loosening affects the glenoid component. Only a small amount of this radiologically visible loosening, however, is clinically relevant. A further complication in the area of the joint socket is increasing glenoid arrosion after shoulder hemiprosthesis, which constitutes the main cause of a surgical revision after hemiprosthesis.

Most frequent complication: prosthesis loosening

The so-called "scapular notching" represents a specific complication of the reverse shoulder prosthesis (Fig. 1.28). This radiological phenomenon describes an osteolysis in the area of the inferior proportion of the joint socket and the scapular neck, resulting from an impingement of the metaglene component at the scapular neck. As a consequence of this osteolysis loosening and breakage of the glenosphere out of the joint socket can occur. Notching can be avoided by an "inferior overlap" of the glenosphere of 0.003–0.005 m.

"Scapular notching": specific complication of reverse shoulder prostheses

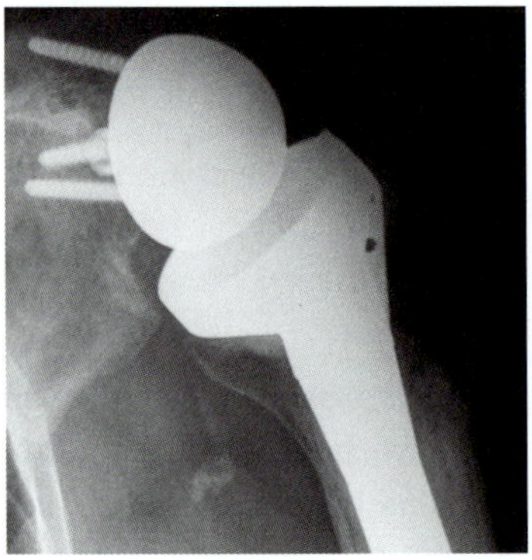

Fig. 1.28: "Scapular notching" on non-contrast radiography.

1.9 Postoperative Rehabilitation

Osseointegration period of the reattached subscapularis tendon determines posttreatment

At implantation of a shoulder prosthesis, an intact subscapular tendon is usually present, which has to be removed and at the end of the operation reattached. The presence of a massive rupture of the rotator cuff is the only exception in the clinical picture of defect arthrography. The post-treatment is mainly determined by the osseointegration period of the reattached subscapularis tendon. Neither the type of prosthesis nor the glenoid replacement usually has any influence on the post-treatment concept.

▸ 1st–14th postop. day

1st Phase: 1st–14th postop. day: passive shoulder joint mobilization
- Immobilization in Gilchrist bandage for four weeks
- Ranges of movement permitted (pain-free without hard impact): 90° flexion, 60° abduction and a **maximum of 10° external rotation**
- Protective measures: ice treatment, lymph drainage, warmth
- Careful passive scapular mobilization

▸ 3rd–6th postop. week

2nd Phase: 3rd–6th postop. week: Development of passive and start of active joint mobility

Goal by the 6th week: reaching for the top of the head and the buttocks without pain
- Removal of the Gilchrist bandage after the 4th postoperative week and start of active mobilization
- Ranges of movement permitted (pain-free without hard impact): 90° flexion, 90° abduction and a **maximum of 20° external rotation**
- Careful active mobilization as well as isometric exercises for scapular stabilizer and rotor cuff (with the exception of the subscapularis muscle)

3rd Phase: 7th–12th postop. week: Development of active joint mobility and strengthening of muscles

▸ 7th–12th postop. week

Goal by the 12th week: painless neck and tying grip

- Free active and passive joint mobilization permitted (pain threshold!)
- Humerus-centered, dynamic, and stabilizing exercises
- Strengthening of the rotator cuff from the 9th week also eccentric
- Scapular stabilization

4th Phase: From the 13th postop. week

▸ From 13th postop. week

- Determining of further procedures and/or return to physical work and sport
- Increasing muscular strengthening of the rotator cuff and scapulo-thoracic musculature, on equipment if necessary
- Dynamic movement exercises to improve coordination

References

Affonso J, Nicholson GP, Frankle MA, Walch G, Gerber C, Garzon-Muvdi J, McFarland EG. Complications of the reverse prosthesis: prevention and treatment. Instr Course Lect 2012;61:157–68.

Bohsali KI, Wirth MA, Rockwood CR. Complications of total shoulder arthroplasty. J Bone Joint Surg Am 2005;88:2279–92.

Boileau P, Avidor C, Krishnan SG et al. Cemented polyethylene versus uncemented metal-backed glenoid components in total shoulder arthroplasty: a prospective, double-blind, randomized study. J Shoulder Elbow Surg 2002;11:351–9.

Boileau P, Walch G. The three-dimensional geometry of the proximal humerus. Implications for surgical technique and prosthetic design. J Bone Joint Surg Br 1997;79:857–65.

Boileau P, Watkinson D, Hatzidakis AM, et al. Neer Award 2005: The Grammont reverse shoulder prosthesis: Results in cuff tear arthritis, fracture sequelae, and revision arthroplasty. J Shoulder Elbow Surg 2006;15:527–40.

Bryant D, Litchfield R, Sandow M, et al. A comparison of pain, strength, range of motion, and functional outcomes after hemiarthroplasty and total shoulder arthroplasty in patients with osteoarthritis of the shoulder. A systematic review and meta-analysis. J Bone Joint Surg Am 2005;87:1947–56.

De Biase CF, Delcogliano M, Borroni M, Castagna A. Reverse total shoulder arthroplasty: radiological and clinical result using an eccentric glenosphere. Musculoskelet Surg 2012;96(Suppl 1):S27–34. Epub 20. 04. 2012.

Gartsmann GM, Roddey TS, Hammerman SM. Shoulder arthroplasty with or without resurfacing of the glenoid in patients who have osteoarthritis. J Bone Joint Surg Am 2000;82:26–34.

Grammont PM, Baulot E. Delta shoulder prosthesis for rotator cuff rupture. Orthopedics 1993;16:65–68.

Jonsson E, Egund N, Kelly I et al. Cup arthroplasty of the rheumatoid shoulder. Acta Orthop Scand 1986;57:542–6.

Karduna AR, Williams GR, Williams JL et al. Glenohumeral joint translations before and after total shoulder arthroplasty. A study in cadavera. J Bone Joint Surg Am 1997;79:1166–74.

Karduna AR, Williams GR, Williams JL et al. Kinematics of the glenohumeral joint: influences of muscle forces, ligamentous constraints, and articular geometry. J Orthop Res 1996;14:986–93.

Kronberg M, Brostrom LA, Soderlund V. Retroversion of the humeral head in the normal shoulder and its relationship to the normal range of motion. Clin Orthop 1990;253:113–7.

Levy O, Copeland SA. Cementless surface replacement arthroplasty (Copeland CRSA) for osteoarthritis of the shoulder. J Shoulder Elbow Surg 2004;13:266–71.

Matsen FA 3rd, Rockwood CA Jr, Wirth MA et al. Glenohumeral arthritis and its management. In Rockwood CA Jr, Matsen FA 3rd, ed. The Shoulder. Philadelphia: Saunders, 1998:840–964.

Murphy LA, Prendergast PJ, Resch H. Structural analysis of an offset-keel design glenoid component compared with a center-keel design. J Shoulder Elbow Surg 2001;10:568–79.

Nho SJ, Frank RM, Verma NN, Romeo AA. Incidence of early development of radiolucent lines in keeled polyethylene glenoid components after total shoulder arthroplasty. Am J Orthop (Belle Mead NJ) 2010;39(7):333–7.

Pearl ML, Volk AG. Coronal plane geometry of the proximal humerus relevant to prosthetic arthroplasty. J Shoulder Elbow Surg 1996;5:320–6.

Pearl ML, Volk AG. Retroversion of the proximal humerus in relationship to prosthetic replacement arthroplasty. J Shoulder Elbow Surg 1995;4:286–9.

Pearl ML. Proximal humeral anatomy in shoulder arthroplasty: Implications for prosthetic design and surgical technique. J Shoulder Elbow Surg 2005; 14(Suppl 1):99–104.

Raiss P, Pape G, Kleinschmidt K, Jäger S, Sowa B, Jakubowitz E, Loew M, Bruckner T, Rickert M. Bone cement penetration pattern and primary stability testing in keeled and pegged glenoid components. J Shoulder Elbow Surg 2011;20(5):723–31. Epub 30. 12. 2010.

Rodosky MW, Bigliani LU. Indications for glenoid resurfacing in shoulder arthroplasty. J Shoulder Elbow Surg 1996;5:231–48.

Walch G, Bacle G, Lädermann A, Nové-Josserand L, Smithers CJ. Do the indications, results, and complications of reverse shoulder arthroplasty change with surgeon's experience? J Shoulder Elbow Surg 2012. Epub ahead of print 22. 2.2012.

Walch G, Boileau P. Shoulder Arthroplasty. Berlin, Heidelberg, New York: Springer, 1999.

Walch G, Edwards TB, Boulahia A et al. The influence of glenohumeral prosthetic mismatch on glenoid radiolucent lines: results of a multicenter study. J Bone Joint Surg Am 2002;84:2186–91.

Wirth MA, Loredo R, Garcia G, Rockwood CA Jr, Southworth C, Iannotti JP. Total shoulder arthroplasty with an all-polyethylene pegged bone-ingrowth glenoid component: a clinical and radiographic outcome study. J Bone Joint Surg Am 2012;94(3):260–7.

Wirth MA, Rockwood CA Jr. Complications of shoulder arthroplasty. Clin Orthop 1994;307:47–69.

I. Schleicher, O. Kilian, R. Schnettler

2 Primary Endoprosthetics of the Hip Joint

2.1 Introduction

In Germany, around 190,000 hip prostheses are implanted per year. The reason for the increasing trend in the quantity of implanted hip prostheses is the longer life expectancy. Hip replacement has become one of the most common operations in orthopedics. With 95 % patient satisfaction, they are among the most successful operations.

Around 19,000 hip prosthesis implants per year

95 % patient satisfaction

In the last few years there has been the tried and tested, but also much that is innovative. Analysis of failures after primary implantation shows the problem of aseptic loosening in over 75 %. Within the first 15p years around 10 % of implants had to be changed because of aseptic prosthesis loosening. More stable fixation techniques for implants using the cementless technique through a change in the surface structures or the hydroxyapatite coating, improved materials in the tribological pairings, the reduction in the polyethylene wear and novel prosthesis design, led to extended durability of the endoprostheses. In the meantime, surgical techniques supported by navigation for better positioning of the implants have become available. Minimally invasive approaches have been established; thus, anatomy-based implantation, even less soft-tissue damage, and faster rehabilitation can be achieved.

Failures after primary implantation: over 75 % aseptic loosening

Extended durability of endoprosthesis and faster rehab through
- more stable fixation
- improved material
- novel prosthesis design
- improved surgical technique

In the perioperative management of the implantation of a hip endoprosthesis, further developments could also be observed. Newly developed medications for the isolated inhibition of coagulation factors may possibly improve thrombosis prophylaxis in high-risk areas, prevent heparin-induced thrombocytopenia, and enable patient-friendly oral application.

New medications for isolated inhibition of coagulation factors

The constant advancements in implants, materials, and designs, but also improvements in surgical techniques and perioperative management, lead to continuous improvement in primary endoprosthetics of the hip joint.

Continual improvement in hip joint primary prosthetics

2.2 Anatomy of the Hip Joint

Anatomy of the hip joint

The hip joint (*articulatio coxae*) is the link between the acetabulum and the femoral head. Two thirds of the femoral head is covered in cartilage. In the middle of the cartilaginous joint surface of the hip joint lies the fovea capitis in which the ligament of the head of the femur joins with the ramus acetabularis (branch of the obturator artery).

Construction of the acetabulum

The acetabulum is hemispheric with a caudal gap, the acetabular notch. Around the edge of the acetabulum lies a fibrocartilaginous ring, the glenoid labrum, which the acetabular ligament bridges in the area of the notch. The acetabulum is covered in cartilage in a half-moon shape in the fossa lunata; the remaining surface is filled with connective and fatty tissue. In the three-dimensional space the acetabulum is at a 45° angle on the side (inclination) in the frontal plane, in the sagittal plane it inclines approx. 20° forward (anteversion). The acetabulum and labrum together cover up to two-thirds of the femoral head. The femoral neck stands on the femoral shaft axis at an angle of around 135° in adults (CCD angle) and in relation to the distal femoral condyles it inclines around 20° forward (antetorsion).

Construction of the articular capsule

The articular capsule originates at the bony edge of the acetabulum and joins the femur in the area of the intertrochanteric line. The articular capsule is strengthened by the iliofemoral, pubofemoral, and ischiofemoral ligaments, which balance and partially impede the movements of the hip joint.

Ball and socket joint with three main axes of movement

The hip joint is a ball and socket joint with three main axes of movement when in the neutral standing position:
- Transverse axis for ante- and retroversion (normal indication anteversion/retroversion = 130°/0°/10°)
- Sagittal axis for the abduction and anteversion (normal indication abduction/adduction = 30–45°/0°/20–30°
- Longitudinal axis for internal and external rotation (normal indication external rotation/internal rotation = 45–50°/0°/30–40°

Muscle groups for movements in the hip joint on the three main axes

The movements in the hip joint on the three main axes are effected by groups of muscles:
- Anteversion: iliopsoas muscle, gluteus maximus muscle, gluteus medius muscle (upper part), rectus femoris muscle, tensor fascia latae muscle.
- Retroversion: gluteus maximus muscle, gluteus medius muscle (lower part)
- Abduction: gluteus maximus (upper half), gluteus medius and minimus muscles
- Adduction: iliopsoas muscle, gluteus maximus (lower half), pectineus muscle, adductor longus, brevis and magnus muscles, gracilis muscle
- Internal rotation: gluteus medius muscle, gluteus minimus muscle, adductor magnus muscle

– External rotation: gluteus maximus (lower half), medius, and minimus muscles (rear part), piriformis muscle, obturator internus muscle, gemelli muscle, quadratus femoris muscle, obturator externus muscle

Stabilization of the hip joint

The braking action of the hyperextension in the hip joint takes place predominantly through band structures, those of the hyperflexion through the dorsal musculature. An important stabilizer of the hip joint is the gluteus medius muscle, which particularly when walking, takes over the main work of stabilization of the pelvis and whose impaired function leads to tilting of the pelvis (Trendelenburg gait). The adductors stabilize medially, the iliopsoas muscle and the rectus femoris ventrally, and the ischiocrural musculature and the rear part of the gluteus maximus dorsally.

Arterial supply of the femoral head

The arterial supply of the femoral head is effected through the lateral and medial circumflex femoral arteries from the femoral artery. For the blood supply of the femoral head the ramus acetabularis, which proceeds in the ligament of the femoral head, has no purpose in adults. This medial circumflex femoral artery runs between the iliopsoas muscle and the pectineus muscle medially and further in the direction of the lesser trochanter. In the adductors two rami branch out, the rami superficialis and profundus, which supply the rear part of the articular capsule. The medial circumflex femoral artery lies topographically beneath the rectus femoris muscle and also divides into two rami: the ramus ascendens, which supplies the front part of the articular capsule, and the ramus descendens the supply of the quadriceps femoris. Because of disruption of vascularization in the articular capsule, lacerations of the articular capsule conceal the danger of femoral head necrosis.

Danger of femoral head necrosis because of disruptions of the articular capsule

2.3 Implant Materials

Biocompatibility and viability of the material are important

Materials for cemented stem prostheses

The materials used for hip endoprosthetics must fulfill the requirements of biocompatibility and viability. Suitable materials currently considered as standard for cement-fixated stem prostheses in chronological order:

- Forged cobalt-chrome-molybdenum (CoCrMo) alloys
- CoCrMo cast alloys
- Forged, highly polished titanium alloys

With the choice of implant materials it should be taken into account that CoCrMo alloys exhibit small amounts of nickel, whereby implant-associated reactions could be triggered in the

With known nickel allergy: cementless implants made of titanium alloys

Materials for cementless prosthesis stems

case of nickel allergy. It is therefore recommended in the case of known nickel allergy to choose cementless implants made of titanium alloys.

For cementless fixated prosthesis stems the following are currently standard:

- Forged cobalt-chrome-molybdenum (CoCrMo) alloys
- Forged titanium alloys

Cemented socket prostheses made of polyethylene

Cementless screwed/press-fit socket with polyethylene inlay

Materials suitable for socket prostheses

Cemented implanted socket prostheses consist of polyethylene (PE). In cementless implantation screwed or press-fit anchored sockets with a polyethylene or ceramic inlay have been introduced. Materials suitable for socket prostheses are in chronological order:

- Pure titanium
- Titanium alloys
- Forged cobalt-chrome-molybdenum (CoCrMo) alloys

Improved osseointegration through surface modification

Material strength of the components is crucial for material wear and the cellular activities triggered by it

Owing to surface roughness as well as a coating of hydroxyapatite improved osseointegration of the stem and socket prosthesis in cementless implantation is achieved.

For the tribological pairing between the prosthesis ball and inlay of the hip socket various materials are available. The strength of the material of the two articulating components is crucial for material wear and the cellular, resorbing activities triggered by them.

Possible tribological pairings

The following tribological pairings exist:

- Metal/polyethylene (metal–PE) – wear rate 150–200 µm per year
- Metal/high-density PE – wear rate 150–180 µm per year
- Al_2O_3/polyethylene (ceramic–PE) – wear rate 50–00 µm per year
- Ceramic/high-density PE – wear rate 30–50 µm per year
- Al_2O_3/Al_2O_3 (ceramic on ceramic) – wear rate 10 µm per year
- Zirconium/zirconium (ceramic on ceramic, Delta prosthesis) – wear rate <10 µm per year; zirconium possesses a greater material strength than aluminum oxide
- CoCrMo/CoCrMo (metal on metal, Metasul) – wear rate <10 µm per year; with a high proportion of molybdenum a new “softer metal property” is achieved, which results in low wear in combination with a fluid-film. Indeed, it is unclear how much of a toxic or carcinogenic effect is exerted by increased metal ion levels.

2.4 Cemented Versus Cementless Implantation

Aims of endoprosthetics

The aim of endoprosthetics, apart from painless functioning and the minimization of wear between the tribological pairings, is the durable fixation of the implants. The fixation of the socket and stem can be cemented or cementless.

For cemented technology bone cement containing antibiotics is applied. The bone cement consists of a polymer powder component (polymethyl methacrylate, PMMA), a monomer fluid component (methyl methacrylate, stabilized by hydroquinone), catalyzers (benzol peroxide) and activators (radicals creator, N,N-dimethyl-p-toluidine, DMPT). By mixing the two component systems, consisting of a powder (polymer) and a fluid (methyl methacrylate), a polymerization process is triggered that leads to the hardening of the cement within 10–12 minutes. Polymerization is linked to a temperature rise (exothermic reaction) in which for each mole of polymerized methacrylates 57 kJ of energy is released. In vivo maximum temperatures within the range 40–46°C are identified at the bone–cement interface.

Cemented technology: bone cement containing antibiotics

Handling of the bone cement

Polymerization is an exothermic reaction
Maximum temperatures in vivo: 40–46°C

In addition to primary instability the principle of cementless fixation is the adhesion of bone at the surface of the prosthesis (osseointegration).

Osseointegration principle of cementless fixation

Primary stability of the implant is achieved by designing for the clamping of the implants, the "press-fit," by stabilizers fixed to the implant, and by the additional fixation of the socket with screws. The aim is the initial prevention of tilting and rotational instabilities after implantation.

Primary stability of the implant influences tilting and rotational instabilities

Secondary stability is guaranteed by osseointegration of the implants, which can be achieved through microporous surface structures or through hydroxyapatite coating.

Secondary stability through osseointegration

The question of whether cemented or cementless implants should be used is controversial. The interaction between implant and/or cement and the surrounding tissue is vital for the durability of the endoprosthesis. It is known that with the cemented implantation technique greater primary stability can be achieved by the cement penetrating into the medullary cavities between the cancellous trabeculae and adjusts to the shape of the endosteal contact area. The osseointegration, i.e. the growth of newly formed bone, is considerably better on a titanium surface than on a cement mantle that exhibits no bioactivity. Increasing osteogenetic activity leads to greater secondary stability with cementless implantation techniques.

Controversial discussion on cemented or cementless implantation

Interaction between implant/cement and soft tissue influences durability

Cemented implantation: greater primary stability

Cementless implantation: greater secondary stability

Long-term results showed no advantage of cementless implantation with regard to durability; thus, the cemented technique being standard is still justified. An advantage of cemented implantation for early rehabilitation is the immediate loading ability of the operated leg. After cementless implantation a non-loading

Cemented technique as standard

Immediate load-bearing ability of the operated leg with cemented implantation

Elderly patients: cemented implantation

Younger patients: cementless implantation

Revision surgery is easier with cementless implantation

Hybrid method as alternative

period of up to six weeks is recommended, while a cemented hip joint endoprosthesis can bear a load straight away. Thus, in older patients cemented implantation and in younger patients cementless implantation of the endoprosthesis is often carried out, although a biological age of about 70–80 years is considered for the decision whether to use cemented or cementless implantation. Another reason for using the cementless implantation technique in younger patients is the high probability of revision surgery over time, which is often simpler to perform with a hip joint endoprosthesis implanted without cement than with a cemented implant. An alternative to the purely cemented or cementless implantation techniques, the hybrid method (cementless socket, cemented stem), is a possibility.

2.5 Cemented Implants

2.5.1 Polyethylene Socket

Cups made of high-molecular-weight polyethylene for cemented implantation technique

Consequences of mis-implantation of the socket

Main problem: loosening of the cemented socket over time

For the cemented implantation technique cups made of high-molecular-weight polyethylene are available. This material demonstrates a low coefficient of friction in various tribological pairings and low abrasion. For the correct positioning of the socket, an abduction angle of between 30° and 55° and an anteversion angle of between 0° and 30° are stated in the literature. A mis-implantation of the socket can lead to iliopsoas impingement, luxations, socket migration and premature loosening by increased polyethylene abrasion. The loosening of a cemented socket over time is still the main problem, with an exponential increase after the eighth postoperative year.

2.5.2 The Cemented Stem

Cemented technique crucial for the durability of the prostheses

Important for the preparation of the medullary cavity: use of a straight stem or anatomical prosthesis

In the field of stem cementing, it could be proven over the last few years that it is not the prosthesis design (Fig. 2.1) but the cementing technique that is crucial to the durability of the prosthesis. An identical shell of cement with no air vents and measuring 0.002–0.003 m thick should be achieved with the implantation.

In the case of cemented techniques of the stem it is important for the preparation of the medullary cavity whether a straight stem prosthesis or an anatomically adapted prosthesis (Tab. 2.1) is used. With the straight stem the medullary cavity is reamed, while with the slightly curved prosthesis the medullary cavity is compressed by careful tapping in. The vacuum cement technique and jet lav-

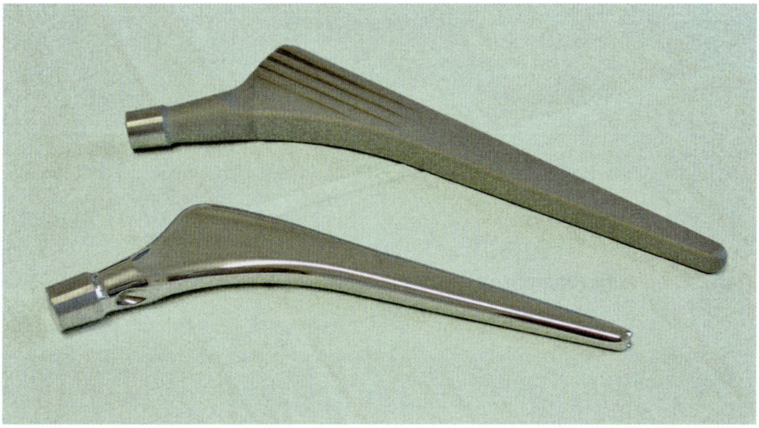

Fig. 2.1: Cementless (above) and cemented stem (below).

Table 2.1: Selection of cemented stems.

	Type of prosthesis	Manufacturer
Straight stem	Bicontact	Aesculap
	Müller straight stem	Smith&Nephew GmbH
	MS-30	Zimmer Germany GmbH
Anatomical stem	Olympia	Biomet
	SP II Lubinus	Link

age, before the cement is introduced into the medullary cavity, are established procedures. To prevent the cement spreading into the whole medullary cavity, cement stoppers made of resorbable material are predominantly used nowadays. But cement stoppers made of polyethylene, or out of corticocancellous chipped bone prepared from the femoral head, are applied.

Cement stopper prevents cement spreading into the whole medullary cavity

2.6 Cementless Implants

2.6.1 Threaded Cup and Press Fit Sockets

Cementless socket systems

As a cementless socket system, conical threaded cups and spherical press-fit sockets have come into use (Figs. 2.2 and 2.3).

Fixation principle of threaded cup sockets

The principle of fixation with the threaded cup is conical milling, screwing in of the socket, and the achievement of primary stability by screw thread geometry.

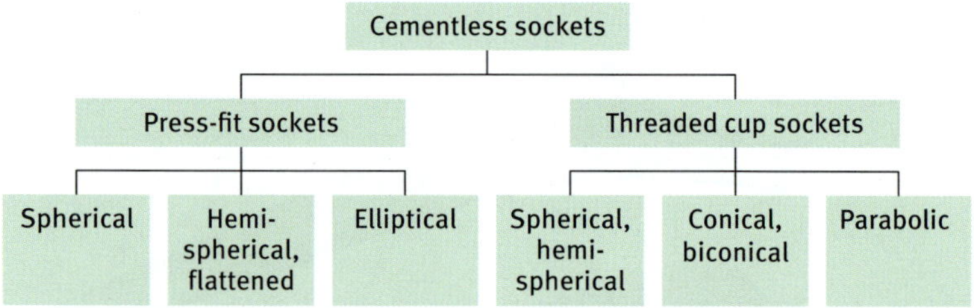

Fig. 2.2: Classification of cementless sockets.

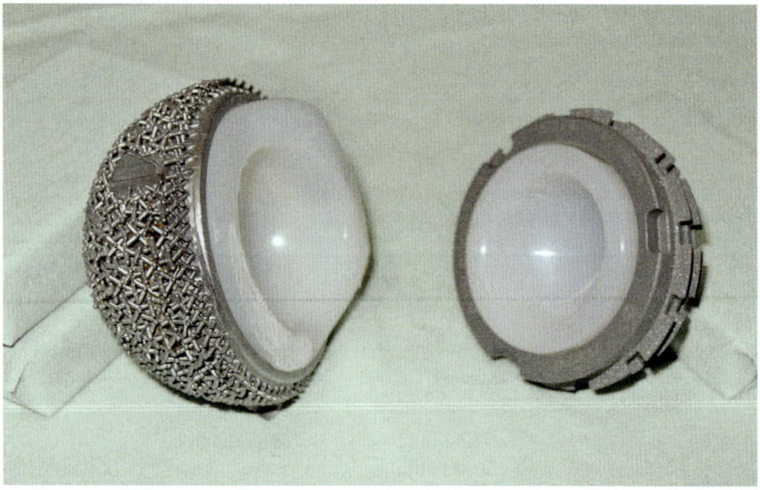

Fig. 2.3: Press-fit socket (left) and threaded cup (right) with polyethylene inlay.

Press-fit implantation
Better osseointegration and lower rates of loosening with spherical sockets

Additional stability through screws, spikes, and pegs

With the press-fit implantation it is spherically, subchondrally milled, and the implant is jammed into the socket holder with an initial load. The contact surface of the spherical socket is larger than with the conical implants. Better osseointegration and lower rates of loosening of the spherical socket are the results of this. Additional stability is guaranteed by the use of screws, spikes or pegs in the direction of the load on the upper edge of the socket so that only push/pull loading, and not tilting, ensues, and an impingement is prevented.

Primary stability of the press-fit sockets by deadlock

Press-fit sockets with hemispherical or elliptical design

The stable fixation of a press-fit socket is achieved by oversizing the socket in comparison to the milling of the acetabulum. The primary stability of the press-fit socket is thus achieved through a deadlock (adhesion and frictionally engaged) in the acetabulum. In contrast to the conical milling with the use of threaded cups the milling of the press-fit socket is hemispherical because of the “half-spherical design” of the acetabulum. The socket also features a hemispherical or elliptical design (Tab. 2.2).

Table 2.2: Selection of hemispherical, flattened hemispherical, and elliptical press-fit sockets.

	Type of prosthesis	Manufacturer
Hemispherical	Trident	Stryker
	Pinnacle	DePuy
	EL socket	Smith&Nephew
	RM Pressfit	Mathys
	Exceed	Biomet
	Continuum	Zimmer Germany
Flattened hemisphere	Allofit	Zimmer Germany
	Plasmacup	Aesculap
	Rimcup	Biomet
Elliptical	TM Cup	Zimmer Germany

Table 2.3: Selection of threaded cup sockets.

	Type of prosthesis	Manufacturer
Hemispherical	Spirofit	DePuy
	Trident	Stryker
Conical	Variall	Zimmer Germany
	Twin 1	Biomet
	SSC Cup	Stemcup
Biconical	Bicon Plus	Smith&Nephew
Parabolic	Hi-Cup	Smith&Nephew
	Parabol	Chiropro

Optimization of the osseointegration of the press-fit socket and the achievement of great secondary stability to prevent rotational and tilting instability is achieved through implants by:

Methods of optimization of osseointegration and an increase in secondary stability

- The crudeness of the structured titanium surfaces (microporous) or by a hydroxyapatite coating applied using the plasma spraying process.
- Additional stabilizers like pegs, spikes, sticks, etc.
- The additional inclusion of screws through boreholes in the socket.

However, it should be stressed that the "press-fit" placement of the socket is definitely the most important factor.

"Press-fit" placement of the socket is the most important form of stabilization

The fixation of threaded cups (Tab. 2.3) is achieved by screw thread geometry. After a conical milling process the implant, made of pure titanium, is screwed into the bony socket holder with self-tapping screws. A flat thread leads to better cutting into the premilled bone, while in the case of a triangular screw thread, it is often a matter of forcing the socket into the bony holder.

Fixation of threaded cup sockets is determined by screw thread geometry

2.6.2 The Bipolar Prosthesis (Dual-Head Prosthesis)

Osteoporosis-related medial femoral neck fracture in older patients main indication for dual-head prosthesis
- Shorter operating times
- Less blood loss
- Immediate full weight-bearing

The main indication for the implantation of a dual-head prosthesis is osteoporosis-related medial femoral neck fractures in older patients. The dual-head prosthesis is a bipolar, femoral hemiprosthesis with an outer ceramic or metal shell, a polyethylene inlay, a cemented stem with a ceramic or metallic head, but with no provision for the acetabulum (Fig. 2.4). The considerably shorter operating times owing to the abandonment of the implantation of a socket and less blood loss in comparison to the "conventional" hip endoprosthesis represent less strain for older patients. The patients can be fully weight-bearing straight away and early rehabilitation can be induced.

Great freedom of rotation and little relative motion

The ceramic or metallic shell and the femoral head prosthesis are self-centering, whereby the centers of rotation of the inner and outer femoral head unit run eccentrically. The outer shell is inclined to assume a vertical position toward the direction of the main loading zone. In this way great freedom of

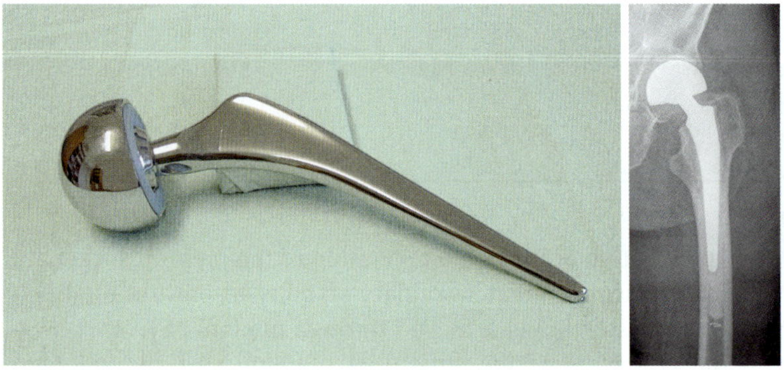

Fig. 2.4: Dual-head prosthesis and radiological features of a dual-head prosthesis.

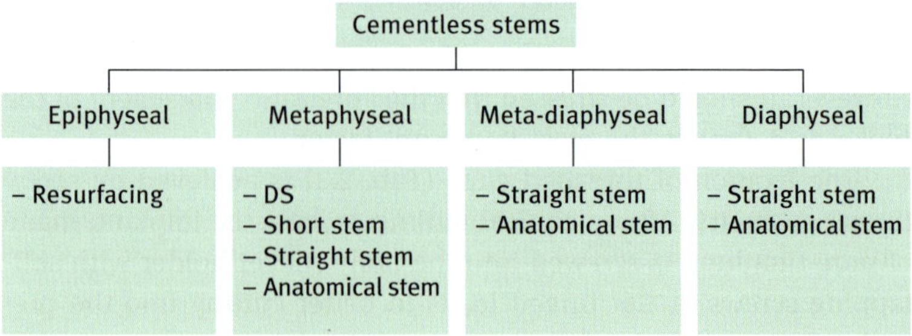

Fig. 2.5: Classification of cementless stems.

rotation and little relative motion between the acetabulum and socket are achieved.

An additional acetabular fracture present at the medial femoral neck fracture or a protruding coxarthrosis is a contraindication to the use of a dual-head prosthesis. Because of the possible complications with protrusion of the artificial femoral head into the pelvis and destruction of the cartilage of the joint socket after a short period, the implantation of a dual-head prosthesis is administered with caution in the younger patient. Rare cases of tumors or femoral head necrosis constitute indications for the implantation of a bipolar prosthesis in the younger patient. An advantage of the dual-head prosthesis consists in the possibility of changing to a unipolar (conventional) hip prosthesis without removal of the femoral components.

Contraindications for dual head prosthesis:
- Additional existing acetabulum fracture
- Protruding coxarthrosis

Tumors, femoral head necrosis are rare indications for implantation of a bipolar prosthesis in the younger patient

2.6.3 Epiphyseal Fixation (Surface Replacement)

As early as the 1970s the surface replacement, e.g., the double cup developed by H. Wagner with a femoral component made of metal or ceramics and with a socket component made of polyethylene came into use. The advantage of this prosthesis system lay in the minimal bone resection. Polyethylene-induced osteolysis, however, led to early loosening and foreign body granuloma; thus, this prosthesis design was soon largely abandoned. The surface replacement ("hip resurfacing"), however, experienced a renaissance about 15–20 years ago. In 1990, a new generation of surface replacements was developed by Derek McMinn of the Royal Orthopaedic Hospital in Birmingham, with the McMinn prosthesis (Birmingham Hip Resurfacing, BHR). In contrast to the conventional hip systems, in resurfacing, the metaphyseal and epiphyseal femoral part remains largely preserved. The anatomical form of the femoral neck, with the caput-collum diaphyseal angle (CCD) and the torsion angle, persists. Minimal resection guarantees unchanged biomechanics with transfer of strength via the femoral neck to the femur and the prevention of stress shielding. Deformity of the proximal femur or a discrepancy in leg length cannot be corrected by resurfacing.

The indication for resurfacing is coxarthrosis in the younger, active patient with no considerable deformation of the joint structures. Secondary coxarthrosis in dysplasia, manifest osteoporosis, coxa vara, bone cysts in the femoral neck, and femoral head necrosis are contraindications for the implantation of a resurfacing sys-

Minimal bone resection advantage of resurfacing

Early loosening and foreign body granuloma through polyethylene-induced osteolysis

McMinn prosthesis new generation of surface replacement

Advantages:
- Unchanged biomechanics
- Prevention of stress shielding

No correction of a deformity of the proximal femur or leg length discrepancy

Coxarthrosis in the younger, active patient indication for resurfacing

Contraindications

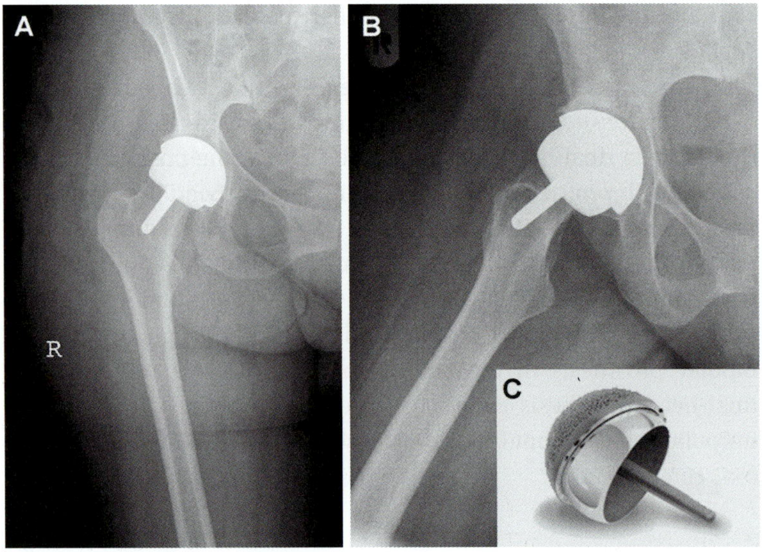

Fig. 2.6: Resurfacing and radiographic findings (Orthopedic Clinic of Thüringen Clinic Saalfeld).

Table 2.4: Selection of resurfacing prostheses.

Prosthesis type	Manufacturer
DUROM® Hip Resurfacing	Zimmer Germany
BHR® Birmingham Hip Resurfacing	Smith&Nephew
ReCap® Resurfacing	Biomet Deutschland

tem. High body mass index (BMI) and prior osteosynthesis of the affected hip joint are considered to be relative contraindications.

Relative contraindications

Construction, material, and design of the resurfacing

Surface replacement (Fig. 2.6, Tab. 2.4) consists of the acetabulum component, which is anchored in the acetabulum using the press-fit (cementless) technique. The sockets are coated with microporous pure titanium or hydroxyapatite in most designs, in order to improve stability and integration of the implants through enhanced osteoconduction. The femoral head shell is implanted using the cemented technique. The hip system exhibits as a special feature very large head diameters, which comply not only with the minimal bone resection, but also with greater stability and a greater range of motion of the prosthesis. The prosthesis design includes abrasion-resistant metal-on-metal tribological pairings (Metasul®); thus, polyethylene-induced osteolysis does not occur.

Surgical approach

Implantation is usually carried out on the lateral side and via a dorsal approach to the hip joint, although extended anterolateral approach to the hip joint is also possible.

As possible complications after implantation of a surface replacement, femoral head fractures, implant-associated impingement by bumping the femoral neck on the socket, luxation and/or subluxation as well as approach-related nerve damage can occur.

Complications of resurfacing after implantation

An Australian study (National Joint Replacement Register 2007) showed an average revision rate after implantation of a resurfacing prosthesis of 2.8 % (0–8.4 %) after 36 months' follow-up. Of 3497 follow-up patients, 50 femoral neck fractures, 12 cases of aseptic socket loosening, 4 cases of aseptic loosening, and 2 infections occurred.

Revision rate after resurfacing implantation approximately 2.8 % in 36 months

The metal-on-metal tribological pairings that are used for resurfacing are currently the focus of discussion. According to a consensus recommendation of the EFORT (European Federation of National Associations of Orthopaedics and Traumatology), the Association of Endoprosthetics (AE) and the organization German Arthrosis Aid, of April 2012, the benefits of the metal-on-metal tribological pairing are low abrasion, few material breakages, low risk of luxation from femoral head size of 0.036 m as well as greater range of motion with large femoral heads. As well as the risk of femoral neck fracture and high bone consumption on the side of the socket, patients are faced with the systemic risks of the spread of metallic products and ions via the circulation, with unknown consequences. Therefore, for all patients with metal-on-metal tribological pairing systematic follow-up with radiography and blood tests with regard to the cobalt level are recommended. In doing this the cobalt value should lie between 2 and 7 µg/l, although the exact threshold is still to be ascertained. If there are abnormalities, revision surgery must be discussed where required. Members of an expert commission are currently carrying out a systematic review of the concentration and level of exposure to metal ions. The result was due at the time of printing.

Metal-on-metal tribological pairings debated

Advantages

Disadvantages

Recommendation: systematic follow-up with radiography and ascertainment of the cobalt level of the blood

Revision if necessary

2.6.4 Metaphyseal Stem Fixation

Femoral neck prostheses (thrust plate prostheses). The femoral neck prosthesis (thrust plate prosthesis) is a cementless hip system with metaphyseal fixation in the preserved femoral neck and proximal femur (Fig. 2.7 and Fig. 2.8). With this hip system, the thrust plate, which rests on the femoral neck, should compensate for the thrust strength and the traction on the plate that is fixed to the proximal femur. Both components are linked to each other with a traction screw that runs through the femoral neck. Requirements for the implantation of a thrust plate prosthesis are the regular

Femoral neck prosthesis (thrust plate prosthesis)

Requirements for implantation

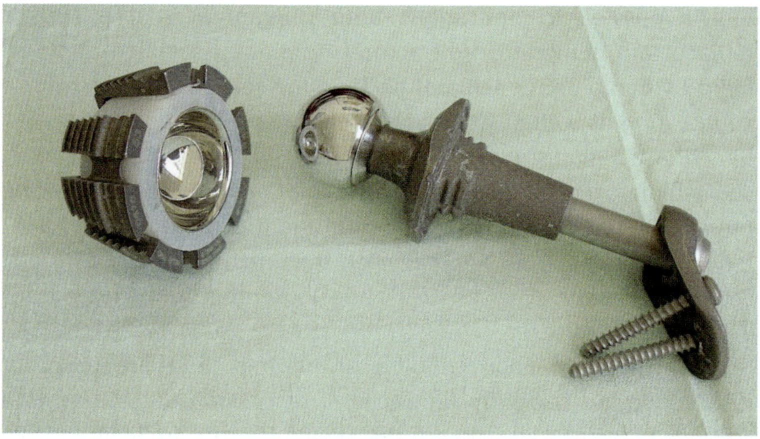

Fig. 2.7: Thrust plate prosthesis with Metasul tribological pairing.

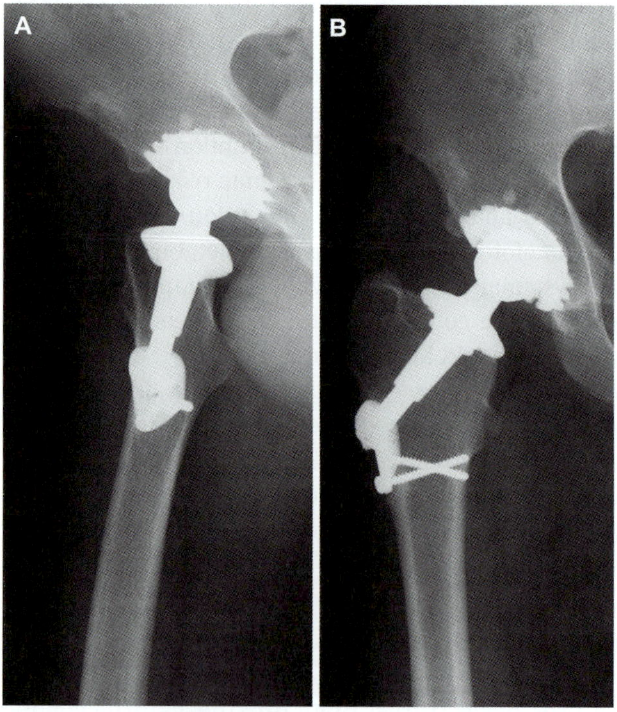

Fig. 2.8: Radiographic findings of a thrust plate prosthesis (Orthopedic Clinic of Thüringen Clinic, Saalfeld).

Contraindication: osteoporotic femoral neck fracture

shape of the femoral neck, a physiological CCD angle (125–130°), and normal bone structure. The osteoporotic femoral neck fracture is a contraindication to the use of this hip system. Because of the high rates of loosening after implantation of a thrust plate prosthesis the question remains whether it is possible for the cancellous bone to withstand the forces that occur. In addition, cortical bone atrophy in the proximal femur was observed. Because of the low bone loss of primary implantation, the requirements for revision endoprosthetics have been amended. Nowadays, the indications for implantation of a thrust plate prosthesis are very narrow. An indication is the coxarthrosis in the "young," active patient with normal bone metabolism and proper morphology of the hip joint.

Lower bone loss with primary implantation requirement for revision endoprosthetics

Indication: coxarthrosis in the "young," active patient

Short stem prosthesis. The Mayo hip stem, implanted without cement, was developed in 1988 in the Mayo Clinic, Rochester. In the meantime even more short stem prostheses from different suppliers have come onto the market. The short stem prosthesis (Tab. 2.5) is based on metaphyseal fixation in the cancellous bone of the proximal femur through multiple points of contact. Because of the low loss of bone mass at implantation the system is suitable for younger patients in whom a revision is very probable. The proximal stem part is conical whereas with the cementless implantation primary stability is achieved and subsidence of the stem prosthesis is prevented. The rotational stability is achieved in metaphyseal fixation by the stem design, with approximation to the anatomical form of the proximal femur.

Short stem prosthesis: metaphyseal fixation in cancellous bone of the proximal femur through multiple points of contact

Because of lower loss of bone mass suitable for implantation in younger patients

With the short stem prosthesis the effect of stress shielding is prevented, a phenomenon that can occur in prosthesis with diaphyseal fixation. With diaphyseal stem fixation decompression of the proximal femur and the area of the trochanteric region can occur, as the load is no longer guided over the bones, but rather over the distally anchored prosthesis stem. The "decompression" of the bone leads to the demineralization and to the slow deformation of the bone because of muscle strain. Consequences of stress shielding may be radiolucent lines, loosening, and periprosthetic fractures. With the use of short stem prostheses an even distribution of stress on the meta- and diaphyseal femoral bone is achieved.

Prevention of stress shielding by short stem prosthesis

Stress shielding: demineralization and deformation of the bone because of muscle strain in diaphyseal fixation

Consequences: radiolucent lines, loosening, periprosthetic fractures

Table 2.5: Selection of thrust plate and short stem prostheses.

Prosthesis type	Manufacturer
Metha Modular Short Stem Prosthesis	Aesculap
CFP Hip Stem	Link
Mayo Short Stem Prosthesis	Zimmer Germany
Nanos Short Stem Prosthesis	Smith&Nephew
Proxima	DePuy
Cut	ESKA
DSP	Sulzer medica

Metaphyseal fixation by special prosthesis design

Prevention of stress shielding

High osseointegration

Metaphyseally anchored straight stem. The metaphyseal fixation of a straight stem (Tab. 2.6) and an anatomical stem (Tab. 2.7) is achieved through the prosthesis design. Additional proximal latitudinal ribs may guarantee even greater rotational stability. The metaphyseally anchored stems do not show any implant–bone contact in the distal portion, thus preventing stress shielding. With the hydroxyapatite coating or sprayed-on titanium alloy, high osseointegration of the stem prosthesis implanted without cement is guaranteed.

Table 2.6: Selection of metaphyseally anchored straight stem prostheses.

Prosthesis type	Manufacturer
GSS System C	Matthys
Bi-Metric	Biomet
Bicontact	Aesculap
CLS® Sportorno® Stem	Zimmer
Enosis	Smith&Nephew

Table 2.7: Selection of metaphyseally anchored anatomical stems.

Type	Manufacturer
CFP Stem	Link
Proxima	DePuy

Meta-diaphyseally anchored straight stem; proximal clamping with distal transfer of strength

Meta-diaphyseally anchored straight stem. The meta-diaphyseally anchored straight stem depends upon a proximal deadlock with a distal transmission of force (Tab. 2.8, Fig. 2.9).

Table 2.8: Selection of meta-diaphyseally anchored standard stems.

Type	Manufacturer
Alloclassic	Zimmer Germany
PPF	Biomet
Corail	DePuy

Meta-diaphyseally anchored anatomical stem:
- Increased primary and rotational stability
- Improved osseointegration
- Prevention of stress shielding

Meta-diaphyseally anchored anatomical stem. Primary stability with optimal adaptation of the prosthesis stem in the bone mass should be achieved by contouring the implant to the anatomy (Tab. 2.9). The anatomical adaptation leads to an even application of force in the proximal femur and increases primary and rotational stability. Improved osseointegration is induced by the roughness of the surface or the hydroxyapatite coating of the proximal portion of the prosthesis. A flattened distal stem tip prevents stress shielding.

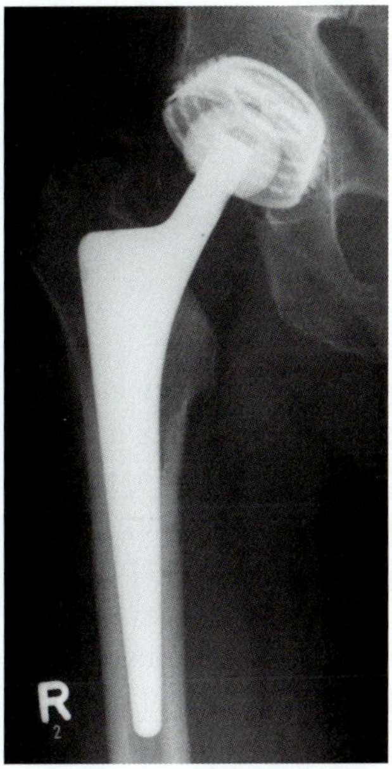

Fig. 2.9: Radiographic findings of a meta-diasphyseally anchored stem and press fit socket.

Table 2.9: Selection of meta-diaphyseally anchored anatomical stems.

Type	Manufacturer
ABG II	Stryker
Cenos	Biomet
AJS	Implantcast
SBG	Smith&Nephew

Diaphyseally anchored stem. Diaphyseally anchored stems are monoblock or modular prostheses and are used not so much in primary implantation as in revision endoprosthetics.

Diaphyseally anchored stems in revision endoprosthetics

2.7 Surgical Approaches

Establishment of minimally invasive approaches in primary implantation

Advantages:
- Protection of soft tissue and muscle

Minimally invasive approaches (minimally invasive surgery, MIS) for the purposes of primary implantation have advanced over the last few years and seem to have become increasingly established. The basic principle of minimally invasive techniques is as little soft tissue trauma as possible in the implantation of the hip endoprosthesis. The advantages of these approaches (e.g., Bauer's transgluteal approach, the dorsal approach) lie in the protection of soft tissue, especially muscle (primarily the abductor musculature), and

▸ Preservation of sensorimotor function

in the preservation of the sensorimotor function, whereby postoperative pain reduction, lower muscular incompetence, and faster early rehabilitation of the patient should be achieved.

Minimally invasive approaches

The following minimally invasive approaches are possible:
- Anterior Smith-Peterson approach
- Anterolateral Watson-Jones approach
- Posterior approach

The fixation methods and implant designs used in minimally invasive techniques

Minimally invasive techniques require specialized instruments and storage facilities. For the implantation standard implants are used with solely cementless fixation, the implantation of a press-fit socket is technically more favorable than the threaded cup; for the stems, short stem prostheses as well as meta- and diaphyseally anchored prostheses are used.

No significant advantages of minimally invasive approach other than less blood loss

A meta-analysis of minimally invasive and conventional approaches was only able thus far to demonstrate slight advantages concerning with blood loss as well as somewhat improved early rehabilitation. With regard to surgery duration, hospitalization of the patient, postoperative pain score, rates of luxation and revision as well as periprosthetic fractures, no significant differences between the various approaches have been able to be established so far. An increased rate of approach-related nerve damage (N. cutaneous femoris lateralis) was established solely for the minimally invasive anterior approach.

2.8 Prophylaxis of Heterotopic Ossification

Incidence of heterotopic ossifications after implantation of a hip joint endoprosthesis >40 %

The incidence of heterotopic ossifications (HO) after implantation of a hip joint endoprosthesis is cited in the literature as being over 40 % without prophylaxis. Risk factors for the formation of ectopic ossifications are the existence of chronic polyarthritis, ankylosing spondyloarthritis, low-dose heparinization, surgery-related factors (approach, intraoperatively dispersed cells) and ossifications after previous endoprosthesis implantation on the contralateral side.

Risk factors

Formation of heterotopic ossifications

Causes of the new bone formation are autoinductive processes induced by the inflammatory stimulus with invasion of stimulated histiocytes, giant cells, and leukocytes into the periarticular soft tissue. By activation of collagenases the collagen matrix degrades and transforms into a vessel-rich crude matrix. Immigrant mesenchymal, pluripotent stem cells distinguish osteoprogenitor cells, which in turn mature into osteoblasts and form heterotopic ossifications. This process is possibly triggered by bone morphogenetic proteins (BMP). The classification of the HO is as follows according to Brooker:

Classification of heterotopic ossifications according to Brooker

- Grade 0: no proof of bone islands
- Grade 1: scattered bone islands in the periarticular soft tissue
- Grade 2: bone/exophytes from the pelvis or femoral head with > 0.01 m gap
- Grade 3: bone/exophytes from the pelvis or femoral head with < 0.01 m gap
- Grade 4: bone bridge/ankylosis between the femoral head and pelvis

Prophylaxis necessary because of high incidence rate

Because of the high incidence rate of heterotopic ossifications prophylaxis is necessary in the implantation of a hip joint endoprosthesis. Effective prophylaxis may be achieved with medication or by localized radiation.

Prophylaxes:
- Nonsteroidal antiphlogistics
- Selective Cox-2 inhibitors

NSAP more efficient, but severe side effects

Medicinally, nonsteroidal antiphlogistics or selective Cox-2 inhibitors are used, whereby prophylaxis administration should take place over 14–21 days (Tab. 2.10). The anti-inflammatory effect affects the inhibitors of prostaglandin synthesis and the reduced proliferation rate of mesenchymal progenitor cells. Studies have shown that nonsteroidal antiphlogistics are more efficient than Cox-2 inhibitors in the prevention of ectopic ossifications (indomethacin is the most efficient), but the side effects such as gastrointestinal symptoms are considerably greater than with Cox-2 inhibitors. The prophylactic application of acetylsalicylic acid and bisphosphonates has been proven in several studies to be ineffective.

Acetylsalicylic acid, bisphosphonates ineffective

High-risk patients: combination of radiation and medical therapy

In high-risk patients radiation and medical therapy can be used as salvage therapy for the purposes of revision surgery.

Table 2.10: Medicinal therapy for the prophylaxis of heterotopic ossifications.

Group	Medication	Application
NSAR	Indomethacin	100 mg/day for 14 days
	Voltaren resinat	150 mg/day for 14 days
	Diclofenac	100 mg/day for 14–21 days
	Ibuprofen	1200 mg/day
	Naproxen	750–1000 mg/day for 8–14 days
	Flurbiprofen	300 mg/day for 14 days
	Acemetacin	200–300 mg/day for 21 days
	Tenoxicam	23–40 mg/day for 14 days
Cox-2 inhibitor	Meloxicam	15 mg/day for 14 days

2.9 Thrombosis Prophylaxis

Surgery-related activation of blood coagulation

The thromboembolic risk factors defined in Virchow's Triad individually contribute to thrombogenesis to an unknown extent. Surgery-related activation of the blood coagulation takes place, the extent of which correlates with the severity of the soft tissue trauma. Because of the different concentrations of thromboplastin in various soft tissues it also depends on the type of soft tissue on which the surgical procedure is carried out. Surgical procedures additionally lead to venous endothelial lesions that may be mechanically, hypoxically or metabolically induced.

Mechanically, hypoxically, or metabolically induced venous endothelial lesions due to surgical procedures

Risk of thrombosis for each patient operated on or immobilized in the longer term

In the communications of the German Association for Surgery, "Recommendations for Stationary and Ambulant Thromboembolism/Prophylaxis," it was established that: "In principle, there is a risk of thrombosis for each patient operated on or immobilized in the longer term."

Elective hip replacement linked to high risk of thrombosis

Incidence of deep vein thrombosis 40–50 %

In keeping with the recommendation of the German Association for Surgery – which was established in 2009 in an S3 guideline – the elective hip replacement belongs to the group with a high risk of thrombosis. While at a medium risk of thrombosis an incidence of deep vein thrombosis (DVT)of 10 to 40 % is indicated, at a high risk of thrombosis it is between 40 and 80 %.

Medical thrombosis prophylaxis, or for contra-indications, intermittent pneumatic compression is necessary

As well as the basic measures such as early mobilization, exercises, guidance on self-exercise, and physical measures (e.g., compression stockings), medical thrombosis prophylaxis should be implemented. For contraindications to medical thrombosis prophylaxis, intermittent pneumatic compression of the foot/calf/thigh should be carried out.

Drug groups for medical thrombosis prophylaxis

For medical thrombosis prophylaxis, the following groups of drugs are available:

- Heparins (unfractionated [UH] and low-molecular-weight fractionated [LMWH])
- Danaparoid
- Isolated inhibitors of factor Xa
- Thrombin inhibitors
- Vitamin K antagonists

ASS (acetylsalicylic acid) should not be used for thrombosis prophylaxis.

Effect of unfractionated heparin

Insufficient protection from deep vein thrombosis, Type II heparin-induced thrombocytopenia

The anti-coagulant effect of unfractionated heparin is based on the activation of anti-thrombosis III vs. thrombin and factor Xa. It is administered subcutaneously at a dosage of 2–3 × 5000 IU/day or 2 × 7500 IU/day. However, unfractionated heparins, in comparison to LMWH, have been proven in meta-analysis to be inferior with regard to the occurrence of deep vein thrombosis, as well as

Table 2.11: Low-molecular-weight heparin (LMWH) for thrombosis prophylaxis in the primary endoprosthetics of the hip joint.

LMWH	Designation
Enoxaparin 40 mg	Clexane 40®
Certoparin sodium	Monoembolex®
Nadroparin calcium	Fraxiparin 0.3®
Dalteparin sodium	Fragmin®
Reviparin	Clivarin®

the incidence of heparin-induced type II thrombocytopenia, and are therefore no longer recommended.

Advantages of low-molecular-weight heparins

In comparison to unfractionated heparin, the administration of LMWH (Tab. 2.11) has the advantage of lower frequency of administration, a lower risk of hemorrhage, and a lower incidence of heparin-induced thrombocytopenia. Indeed, with limited renal function, there is a cumulative risk. The prophylaxis should be started on the eve of the operation and continued for 20–35 days.

Heparin-induced thrombocytopenia Types I and II

After administration of low-molecular-weight heparin, the formation of heparin-induced thrombocytopenia (HIT) may occur. Distinction is made between Type I HIT, which proceeds asymptomatically and does not require treatment, and a symptomatic, life-threatening Type II HIT. With Type II HIT an immunological reaction against the LMWH-induced heparin platelet factor 4 complex takes place, with activation of the platelets and plasma coagulation system. The risk of symptomatic heparin-induced thrombocytopenia after LMWH administration is cited as being 0.05–6.5 %.

Risk: 0.05–6.5 %

Diagnosis of heparin-induced Type II thrombocytopenia

The diagnosis of Type II HIT comprises three criteria:
- Heparinization (unfractionated or low-molecular-weight)
- Presence of thrombocytopenia
- Proof of heparin platelet factor 4 complex using ELISA

HIT correlates with a higher risk of deep vein thrombosis

Heparin-induced thrombocytopenia correlates with a high risk of deep vein thrombosis after an endoprosthetics operation. For this reason, a regular check of the platelet count should be carried out up to at least the 14th day after implementation. In patients at risk of HIT II and planned implantation of a hip joint endoprosthesis, neither unfractionated nor low-molecular-weight heparin must be administered. The anticoagulation occurs with use of the heparinoid danaparoid sodium (Orgaran®), which inhibits antithrombin-mediated factor Xa, or with the recombinant hirudin compound lepirudin (Refludan®; Tab. 2.12).

No unfractionated or low-molecular-weight heparin for at-risk patients

Fondaparinux (Arixtra®) is an antithrombin-mediated factor Xa inhibitor, which, at a dosage of 2.5 mg/day s.c. is very effective,

Table 2.12: Medical thrombosis prophylaxis with HIT II.

Group	Designation	Administration
Danaparoid sodium	Orgaran®	750 IU s.c. twice a day for a maximum of 14 days
Lepirudin	Refludan®	0.4 mg/kg body weight i.v. as a bolus, also 0.15 mg/kg body weight per hour i.v.

Fondaparinux reduced thromboembolisms, but increased hemorrhagic complications

but it should also be given at a reduced dose for renal insufficiency. In meta-analysis it proved to be more effective compared with LMWH in the reduction of thromboembolisms, but there was an increase in hemorrhagic complications, which is why fondaparinux should be given six hours after an operation at the earliest.

New antithrombotic therapy by specific inhibition of individual enzymes of the coagulation cascade

A new era of antithrombotic medical therapy was ushered in with the specific inhibition of individual enzymes of the coagulation cascade. Advantages compared with the previous prophylaxis with LMWH are the independence of antithrombin 3, the oral form of administration, and the discontinuation of therapeutic monitoring. Currently, two medications are available. Dabigatran (Pradaxa®) is a direct thrombin inhibitor.

No significant difference between oral and subcutaneous administration

A comparable double-blinded study did not result in any significant difference in the prevention of venous thromboembolisms after implantation of a hip endoprosthesis between orally administered dabigatran and subcutaneously administered enoxaparin 40. The recommended dose is 220 mg, whereby it should be started 1–4 hours after the operation at only half the dose, and additionally a reduction in renal sufficiency must be considered.

Rivaroxaban with significantly lower occurrence of deep vein thrombosis

Rivaroxaban (Xarelto®), a direct factor Xa inhibitor (Tab. 2.13), showed in several studies a significantly lower occurrence of deep vein thrombosis in comparison to enoxaparin after implantation of a hip endoprosthesis. The risk of hemorrhage showed no signifi-

Table 2.13: Oral thrombosis prophylaxis with factor X and factor II inhibitors.

Group	Designation	Administration
Dabigatran	Pradaxa®	From 1 to 4 hours postoperatively 1 capsule (110 mg); from 1st p.o. day 220 mg/day for 10 days
Rivaroxaban	Xarelto®	From 1 to 4 hours postoperatively 1 capsule (10 mg); from 1st p.o. day 10 mg/day for 5 weeks

Table 2.14: Recommended intervals between medical thrombosis prophylaxis and spinal puncture.

Medication	Last dose before puncture/catheter	Next dose after puncture/catheter removal
UH	4 h	1 h
LMWH	12 h	2–4 h
Danaparoid	If possible no spinal anesthesia or single-shot	
Fondaparinux	36–42 h	6–12 h
Hirudin	8–10 h	2–4 h
Vitamin K antagonists	INR <1.4	Possible immediately

cant differences when both substances were used. The medication should be started at 10 mg six hours after the operation.

Vitamin K antagonists (warfarin, phenprocoumon) inhibit the synthesis of vitamin K-dependent coagulation factors II, VII, IX, and X. The start of the effect is delayed and the dosage has to be tailored individually. In addition, vitamin K antagonists were shown in the evaluation of several studies to be less effective than LMWH with regard to the risk of thrombosis; thus, they are not recommended for medical thrombosis prophylaxis.

Vitamin K antagonists not recommended for medical thrombosis prophylaxis

Important: interval between medical thrombosis prophylaxis and spinal puncture

Because nowadays hip prosthesis implantations are carried out under spinal anesthesia, it is imperative to take into account the interval before the introduction of local anesthesia and catheter removal (see Tab. 2.14).

In summary, in elective hip operations medical thrombosis prophylaxis may be carried out with low-molecular-weight heparins (LMWH), fondaparinux, dabigatran or rivaroxaban. The latter three are particularly recommended if there is early occurrence of heparin intolerance. If LMWH is used, it can be started on the eve of the operation, fondaparinux or rivaroxaban can given six hours after the operation at the earliest, dabigatran 1–4 hours after the operation with half of the dose to be used afterward. The medical prophylaxis should be implemented for 28–35 days.

For elective hip operations medical thrombosis prophylaxis with low-molecular-weight heparins, fondaparinux, dabigatran or rivaroxaban

2.10 Autologous Transfusions

The average blood loss in the primary implantation of a hip joint endoprosthesis, no matter which system is used, is cited as being 900 ± 500 ml intraoperatively and 1150 ± 450 ml postoperatively (total blood loss 2050 ± 950 ml). In a planned implantation the transfusion of homologous stored blood should be avoided, if pos-

Average blood loss: intraoperatively 900 ± 500 ml, postoperatively 1150 ± 450 ml

Avoidance of the transfusion of homologous stored blood

Methods of replacing autologous blood components

sible. To replace autologous blood components various methods are available:

- Autologous donation
- Fresh frozen plasma (FFP) donation
- Normovolemic hemodilution
- Mechanical autotransfusion from intraoperatively salvaged blood

Removal of autologous blood at around 4–6 weeks before the planned implantation

Probability of administration of autologous blood reserves of around 5 %

Efficiency of hemodilution dependent upon end hematocrit value and dilution gradient

Contraindications to intraoperative mechanical autotransfusion of salvaged blood: malignancies, septic lesions

Autotransfusion of salvaged blood one of the most common transfusion methods

The removal of autologous blood takes place at around 4–6 weeks before the planned implantation. Because of the limited storage period, the timing of the operation is established with the start of autologous donation. The possible weakness of the patient through prior autologous donation is also to be taken into account. In patients with pre-existing cardiac conditions in particular this is a factor that should be considered. The most common method of storage after autologous blood removal is the processing of erythrocyte concentrates (EC) and plasma (FFP). The probability of the administration of autologous blood stores being necessary in primary implantation is around 5 %. Alternatives to autologous blood donation are the use of acute hemodilution and the mechanical autotransfusion of intraoperatively salvaged blood. The efficiency of hemodilution is dependent on the end hematocrit value and dilution gradient. The blood components gained through hemodilution may not be retransfused into the patient until the end of the operation because of the coagulation factors present in them. Because only malignancies and septic lesions count as contraindications to an intraoperative medical autologous transfusion of salvaged blood, this method is among the most commonly used methods of transfusion of autologous blood components in primary implantation.

2.11 Rehabilitation after Implantation of a Hip Joint Endoprosthesis

Differing management of early postoperative rehabilitation

Early postoperative rehabilitation in an acute care clinic after implantation of a hip joint endoprosthesis is not managed in a standardized manner, but is often dependent upon the decision of the surgeon. The most important criterion for the possibility of immediate weight-bearing is the primary stability of the implants. The considerable differences in after-care arise from the fact that the information in the literature ranges from immediate weight-bearing without using two underarm crutches to a six-week period of non-weight-bearing or partial weight-bearing with the three-point gait.

The aim of early rehabilitation is the improvement of the hip function and the simultaneous stabilization of the hip through:

Methods of early rehabilitation to improve the articular function and stabilization of the joint

- Prevention of muscular deficiency through active exercise
- Pain relief through muscle-stimulating measures
- Improvement of the joint function (passive and active exercise, use of a CPM device with hip flexion less than 90°, then the ergometer)
- Improvement of the joint function through manual stretching of the contracted articular capsule (thermal, stretch massage therapy)
- Gait training with partial weight-bearing (three-point gait) up to full weight-bearing (four-point gait)
- Prevention of a Duchenne or Trendelenburg limp through efficient gait training with full weight-bearing on the operated leg as early as possible and omission of underarm crutches
- Training in the activities of daily living (ADL)

Rehabilitation on the day of the operation

On the day of the operation the operated leg is positioned in a flat foam brace, cryotherapy is used, and isometric tension exercises are started.

Rehabilitative measures on the first postoperative day

Rehabilitative measures on the first postoperative day are:
- Active extending and flexing of the ankle to improve the blood circulation (thrombosis prophylaxis)
- Isometric tension exercises for the hip flexor and extensor
- Respiratory exercises
- Sitting on the bed

Within 24 hours the patient should already have stood by the bed.

Physiotherapy exercises from the third to the sixth postoperative day

On the third to sixth postoperative days the physiotherapy exercises begin, which make a crucial contribution to the swift recovery of physiological movement sequences in early rehabilitation:
- Extension and flexion in the hip joint, first passively, then actively
- Isometric tension exercises for the internal rotators
- Gait training

Gait training

Through gait training in particular a physiological gait pattern should be achieved as soon as possible. Depending on the loading capacity of the operated leg various gait patterns are possible with the aid of underarm crutches:

Two-point gait

- Two-point gait: the underarm crutches are simultaneously placed diagonally (right leg – left crutch, left leg – right crutch) for axial loading with half of the body weight

Three-point gait

Four-point gait

- Three-point gait: the affected leg is positioned forwards between two underarm crutches just touching the ground or with partial weight-bearing
- Four-point gait: the underarm crutches are positioned diagonally (right left – left crutch, left leg – right crutch) one after another with a delay

Steady gait pattern at discharge

On discharge from the acute care clinic after around 14 days for a normal course (minimum stay 4 days, maximum 21 days) the patients should show a steady gait pattern.

Continuation of rehabilitation after discharge

The continuation of rehabilitation after discharge from the acute care clinic can take place in within the services of the statutory medical or pension insurance institutions with stationary follow-up treatment, within employer's liability insurance association-funded stationary postoperative management or in extended ambulant rehabilitation. Stationary rehabilitation lasts around three weeks; it is necessary until an individually optimal gait pattern with full weight-bearing is achieved.

Radiological follow-up

Radiological follow-up is recommended in the early postoperative period as well as at 3, 6, and 12 months.

References

Grochola LF, Habermann B, Mastrodomenico N, Kurth A. Comparison of periprosthetic bone remodelling after implantation of anatomic and straight stem prostheses in total hip arthroplasty. Archives of Orthopaedic and Trauma Surgery 2008;4:383–92.

Smith TO, Blake V, Hing CB. Minimally invasive versus conventional exposure for total hip arthroplasty: a systematic review and meta-analysis of clinical and radiological outcomes. Int Orthop 2011;35:137–42.

C. Merle, J. Herre, P.R. Aldinger

3 Endoprosthetics of the Knee Joint

3.1 Introduction

The primary replacement of the knee joint is among the most commonly performed surgical interventions in orthopedics and trauma surgery, and represents the gold standard in the treatment of advanced osteoarthritis of the knee. In Germany, more than 160,000 implantations are carried out each year, with a tendency to increase. Through the continual development of prosthesis design and materials, as well as the standardization of the implantation technique, in the meantime, very good long-term results have been presented, with revision-free durability of over 90 % after 15 years. Since the initial experimental implantation of a knee joint hinge prosthesis made of ivory by Themistocles Gluck in 1890, the knee joint endoprosthesis has achieved a high stage of development, especially with the progress of the last 15 years. There is a multitude of prosthesis designs available, which enable individualized patient care, even in complex initial situations. Thus, the choice of a suitable implant system, in connection with a precise indication status and an exact surgical technique, is of crucial significance in achieving a good long-term result. The current prosthesis designs are manufactured out of special metal alloys (CrCoMo). This sliding surface consists of polyethylene (PE), with some manufacturers of by now ultra-high molecular weight polyethylene (UHWPE), which displays in similar attempts comparatively better wear qualities and thus allows better long-term results to be expected.

Gold standard in the treatment of advanced osteoarthritis

More than 160,000 primary implantations a year

Revision-free 15-year durability of more than 90 %

Multitude of prosthesis designs

Individualized patient care even in complex initial situations

Prosthesis designs made of special metal alloys (CrCoMo)

In the last few years various surface improvement treatments and coatings have been clinically tested (titanium coating, ceramization); indeed, until now, in comparison to the classic metal alloy (CrCoMo), no advantage of these expensive procedures has been proven.

No advantage of surface improvements, coating

3.2 Anatomical and Biomechanical Principles

The knee joint (Fig. 3.1) is the largest in the human body and is subject to a high mechanical load. It is divided into joint parts (compartments) with a total of six joint surfaces:

- Articulatio femoropatellaris (femoropatellar compartment)
- Articulatio femorotibialis medialis (medial femorotibial compartment)

Knee joint the largest joint in the body; with high mechanical load

Joint parts of the knee joint

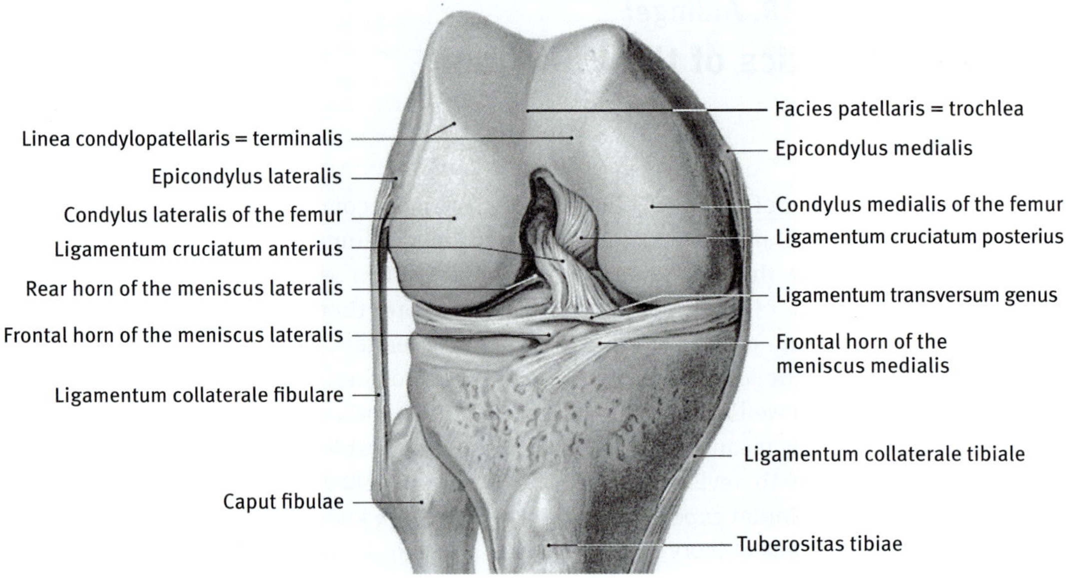

Fig. 3.1: Anatomy of the knee joint, ventral view.

– Articulatio femorotibialis lateralis (lateral femorotibial compartment)

Joint stability through complex interaction of passive and active stabilizers

The stability of the knee joint is guaranteed by a complex interaction of passive (articular capsule, collateral ligaments, cruciate ligaments, retinacula, menisci) and active (quadriceps femoris muscle, ischio-crural musculature, popliteus muscle) stabilizers.

Mikulicz line – mechanical leg axis

Varus or valgus malalignment if the Mikulicz line is medialized or lateralized

With a neutral leg axis the weight-bearing line (Mikulicz line, mechanical leg axis) in the frontal level from the midpoint of the femoral head to the midpoint of the talar dome through the medial part of the eminentia intercondylaris. If the Mikulicz line is medialized or lateralized, it is called varus or valgus malalignment. The anatomical leg axis, which resulted from the angle of the intramedullary femur and tibial axes, forms a valgus angle of approximately 5–10°. Physiologically, the joint line of the knee joint falls in the coronal plane from lateral to medial by approximately 3°; the joint surface of the tibia tilts into the sagittal plain by about 5–15° dorsally (slope) (Fig. 3.2).

Movement sequence of the knee joint as a complex roll-slide-rotate movement

The movement sequence of the knee joint overlaps the reproduction of a simple hinge joint. It is a matter of a complex roll-slide-rotate movement with ventrodorsal translation of the femur towards the tibia in increasing flexion of the knee joint (rollback mechanism).

Because the medial tibia plateau is concave, while the lateral tibia plateau shows a convexity, the smaller lateral femoral condyle

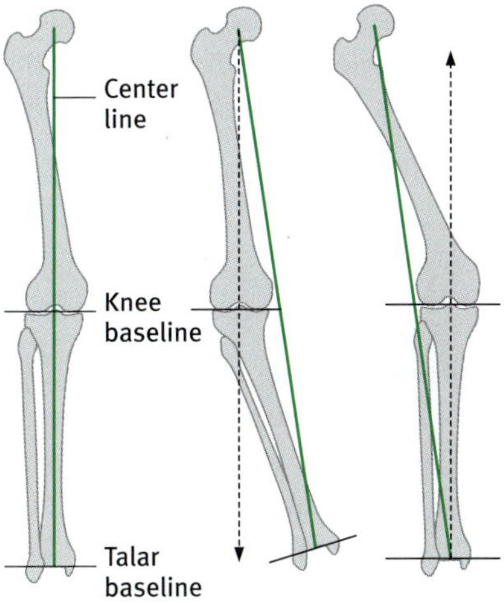

Fig. 3.2: Axial ratios of the lower extremity, a.p.: physiological leg axis (left), varus deformity (center), and valgus deformity (right).

slides further dorsally than the medial, so that with increasing flexion of the knee joints additional internal rotational motion of the tibia occurs. This corresponds to the principle of "medial pivot," (English "pivot" = center of rotation). Furthermore, a limited scope for an active rotation of the knee joint is possible, through the relaxing of the cruciate ligaments in flexion. During the end phase of the extension by pulling the anterior cruciate ligament and the tractus iliotibialis the external rotation of the tibia as opposed to the femur (end-range rotation) occurs, which enables maximal stabilization of the joint when stretching by tensing of the capsule and the collateral ligaments. End-range rotation is reversed by the tensing the popliteus muscle during the early phase of flexion.

Movement sequence of the knee joint

3.3 Gonarthrosis

3.3.1 Epidemiology

Arthrosis of the knee joint is among the most common forms or arthrosis. Its prevalence increases with age and is higher in the female than in the male population. Studies start at a prevalence of symptomatic gonarthrosis in over-55-year-olds of approximately 12.5 %. The prevalence of radiologically manifest gonarthrosis in the over 50s lies at up to 68 %. Estimates of the incidence of gonarthrosis vary dramatically (45–900 new cases per 100,000 life-years). With regard to the future demographic development in Germany the "collective disease arthro-

Knee joint arthrosis is one of the most common forms of arthrosis

Prevalence increases with age

Prevalence higher in women

High expectations of results

Increasing requirement for activity into old age

sis" will gain increasing importance as a socio-medical and economic problem. This is in the face of the high expectations of patients of the result of a surgical intervention as well as an increasing requirement for activity into old age.

3.3.2 Etiology and Classification

Primary arthrosis of largely unknown cause

Secondary arthrosis a consequence of a congenital or acquired joint defect

Arthrosis is divided clinically on the basis of its etiology into two groups: primary (idiopathic) arthrosis, the cause of which is largely unknown, is distinguished from secondary forms of arthrosis, which manifest as a consequence of a congenital or acquired joint defect (Table 3.1). The ratio of primary gonarthrosis to secondary forms of arthrosis is 2 : 1.

Primary gonarthrosis probably has multifactorial causes

Risk factors

Contrary to earlier assumptions that primary gonarthrosis is an age-related, purely mechanical deterioration of the most frequently loaded articular surfaces, it is now assumed that it has multifactorial causes. Risk factors that promote the occurrence and/or progression of primary arthrosis are increasing age, female gender, being overweight, as well as increased bone density. A genetic predisposition also appears to be etiologically relevant.

Table 3.1: Important causes of secondary gonarthrosis.

Trauma	**Traumatic lesions of the internal structure of the knee (e.g., cartilage, meniscus, cruciate ligaments)**
	Intra-articular fractures Free-floating fragments Post-traumatic instability
Dysplastic joint disorder	Condylar hypoplasia
Axial malalignment	Genu varum/valgum congenital or acquired Extra-articular fractures
Inflammatory disease	Bacterial arthritis Rheumatoid arthritis
Metabolic disease	Hyperuricemia Chondrocalcinosis Hemochromatosis Ochronosis
Coagulopathy	Hemophilia
Other causes	Osteochondrosis dissecans Aseptic osteonecrosis (Ahlbäck's disease) Marfan syndrome Ehlers-Danos syndrome Neuropathic joint disorder (arthropathy)

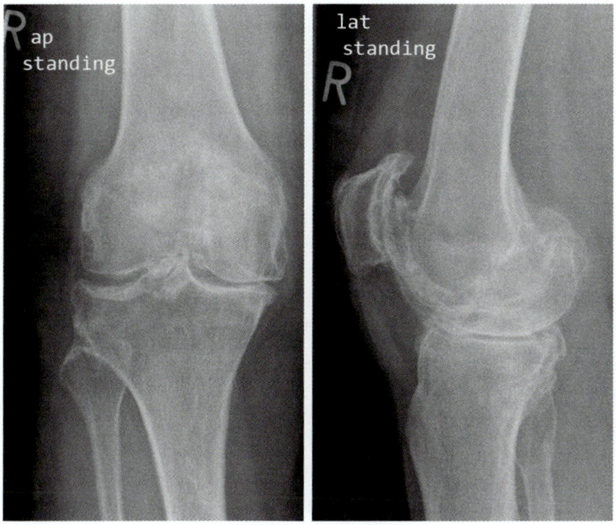

Fig. 3.3: Pangonarthrosis, a.p. and lateral.

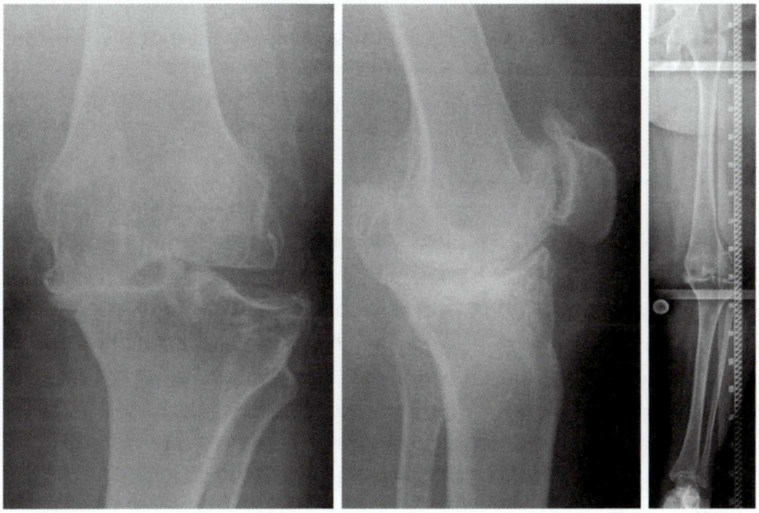

Fig. 3.4: Varus gonarthrosis, a.p. lateral, long leg view.

Morphological distinction of pangonarthrosis from varus gonarthrosis, valgus gonarthrosis, and femoropatellar arthrosis

Morphologically, pangonarthrosis (Fig. 3.3), with distinct degenerative changes in all three knee joint compartments, is distinguished from varus gonarthrosis (Fig. 3.4), valgus gonarthrosis (Fig. 3.5), and femoropatellar arthrosis. In varus and valgus gonarthrosis the medial or lateral compartment is predominantly affected, which through the unilateral decrease in the joint space, leads to a corresponding axial deformity of the lower extremity. Isolated arthrosis

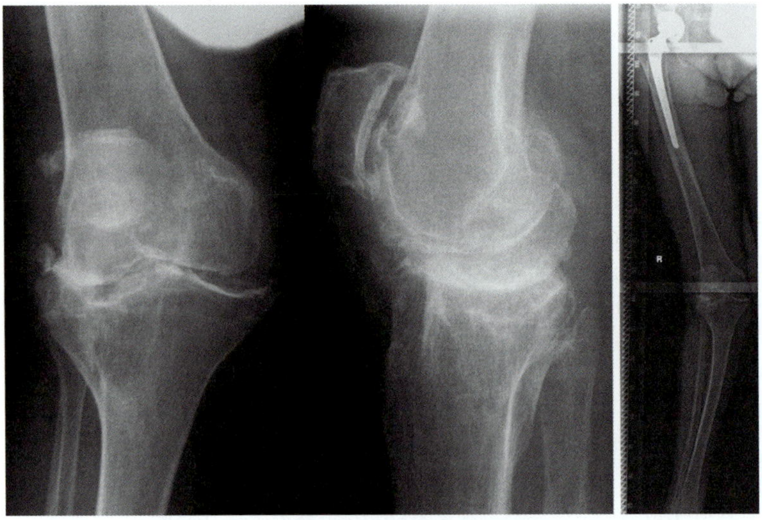

Fig. 3.5: Valgus gonarthrosis with lateral tibial defective zone, a.p., lateral, long leg view.

of the femoropatellar compartment is rarer and affects predominantly the female gender. The extent and localization of the arthritic changes influence the therapeutic concept, the choice of implant, the after-care, and the prognosis of the surgical intervention.

3.3.3 Clinic

Gonarthrosis: pains in the knee joint area
Pain when walking, feeling of instability, load-induced swelling tendency typical of arthrosis

Patients with gonarthrosis predominantly complain of pains in the knee joint area that are initially load-related and also described as rest or night pain in the advanced stages. Additionally, a typically arthritic warm-up pain, a feeling of instability, and a load-induced swelling tendency are often present. Pain-free walking distance is increasingly limited and loads are avoided, which means a loss of quality of life for the patient.

Anamnesis: previous therapeutic measures

Anamnesis determines specific previous conservative (physiotherapy, pain medication) and invasive (intra-articular injections, previous surgery) therapeutic measures. The clinical analysis of the knee joint should take the following aspects into consideration:

Parameters of the clinical analysis of the knee joint

- Gait pattern of the patient, any aids needed
- Evaluation of the leg axis and a possible difference in leg length
- Range of movement according to the neutral zero method
- Stability test
- Evaluation of patella tracking
- Orienting analysis of the contiguous joints, especially the hip joint

- Ascertainment of neurovascular status
- Signs of infection

The differential diagnosis takes a multitude of intra- and/or extra-articular causes of pain into consideration; thus, it should be observed that some of the following differential diagnoses can also underlie secondary arthrotic changes:

Many intra- and/or extra-articular causes of pain

Possible differential diagnoses

- Intra-articular pathologies (e.g., meniscal lesions, osteochondrosis dissecans, osteonecrosis)
- Periarticular pathologies (e.g., bursitis, insertional tendinopathy)
- Diseases of the hip joint (e.g., coxarthrosis, pain radiating into the knee joint)
- Inflammatory diseases (e.g., diseases of the rheumatism spectrum, bacterial arthritis)
- Metabolic diseases (e.g., chondrocalcinosis, hyperuricemia)
- Angiopathy (e.g., PAOD, claudicatio intermittens)
- Neurological diseases (e.g., radicular/pseudoradicular syndrome, neuropathy)
- Neoplasias (e.g., primary tumors, metastases, PUNS)

3.3.4 Imaging Diagnostics

To diagnose gonarthrosis with certainty an X-ray of the affected knee joint in the standing position in two planes (a.p. and lateral), as well as a tangential patellar X-ray in 30° flexion, is sufficient. For special problems other views may be required. For analysis of the leg axis a long leg X-ray (a.p.) should be produced. If a patellar pathology is at the orefront, tangential X-rays at 30°, 60°, and 90° flexion of the knee joint are informative. With unicompartmental arthrosis varus and valgus stress radiograph and/or a p.a. Rosenberg view (in a posterolateral defect zone) may gather additional information for the evaluation of the extent of cartilage damage.

Diagnosis of gonarthrosis with certainty by means of X-rays of the affected knee joint

Other X-rays may be necessary for special problems

Other imaging procedures (MRT, CT, ultrasound, skeletal scintigraphy) are reserved for special problems and play a secondary role in the diagnosis and treatment planning for gonarthrosis.

Further imaging procedures for special problems

3.4 Indications and Contraindications

The indication for implantation of a knee joint endoprosthesis may be obtained in the case of advanced, clinically and radiologically manifest joint destruction with treatment-resistant pain in spite of extensive conservative and if necessary invasive measures, and

Indication: advanced, manifest joint destruction with treatment-resistant pain

Contraindications to endoprosthetic intervention

consideration of the patient's quality of life. Contraindications of an endoprosthetic intervention are:
- Acute or chronic infections of the knee joint
- Skin lesions in the area of the operating field
- Ulcus cruris
- Thrombosis
- Nail bed infections
- Vascular disorders

3.5 Surgical Goals

Surgical goals:
- Freedom from pain
- Adequate stability of the operated joint
- Good every-day functioning

The main goal of endoprosthetic knee joint replacement is freedom from pain for the knee joint, which can be achieved in a substantial number of the patients operated on. Moreover, adequate stability of the operated joint is of vital importance, because postoperative instability not only damages patient satisfaction, it also limits the lifespan of the implant by causing additional wear and premature loosening. Mobility with flexion of over 100° at full extension is required for good every-day functioning. Very often, a vital improvement in the patient's quality of life through pain reduction (>90 %) and improvement in function can be achieved. In comparison to the total endoprosthetic care of the hip joint, in which nearly all patients demonstrate high rates of satisfaction, postoperative patient satisfaction after knee prosthesis is significantly lower at around 85 %.

Patient satisfaction after knee joint prosthesis approximately 85 %

3.6 Risk and Success Factors

Factors regarding the quality of results after implantation of a knee joint endoprosthesis

The quality of results after implantation of a knee joint endoprosthesis depends on various factors:
- Patient age at the time of implantation
- Patient activity in dealing with endoprosthetic joint replacement, compliance
- Co-morbidities
- Design of the implants
- Tribological features of the implant components
- Fixation mode of the implants
- Adequate patient selection and indication setting
- Surgical technique: correct alignment of the implant components, reliable fixation, creation of even soft-tissue tension, precise patellar tracking
- Surgeon

3.7 Preoperative Measures

In most endoprosthetic interventions it is a matter of a surgical procedure of an elective nature; thus, the preoperative minimization of risk is vitally important. Initially, co-morbidities of the patient should be elicited in order to be able to carry out in cooperation with the supervising internist and anesthesiological specialists an extensive estimation of the surgical risks and introduce appropriate therapeutic measures. Preoperatively, an up-to-date laboratory with coagulation and inflammation parameters (CRP) is required.

Preoperative risk minimization very important

Co-morbidities

Up-to-date laboratory with coagulation and inflammation parameters

3.7.1 Surgical Planning

The preoperative planning is an essential aspect of the standard procedure in endoprosthetic interventions. X-rays of the knee joint in two planes, a long leg X-ray as well as a tangential patellar X-ray constitute the basic radiological diagnosis, in order to be able to evaluate the leg axis and the "patella tracking." With the aid of the preoperative X-rays, the prosthesis design, size, the degree of coupling, and resection planes can be ascertained taking into consideration the findings of the clinical analysis. In bicondylar resurfacing the size determination of the femoral components on the lateral X-ray with the aid of the a.p. diameters of the condyles, the size of the tibial components is determined, taking into considera-

Preoperative planning an essential part of the standard procedure in endoprosthetic interventions

Basic radiological diagnosis

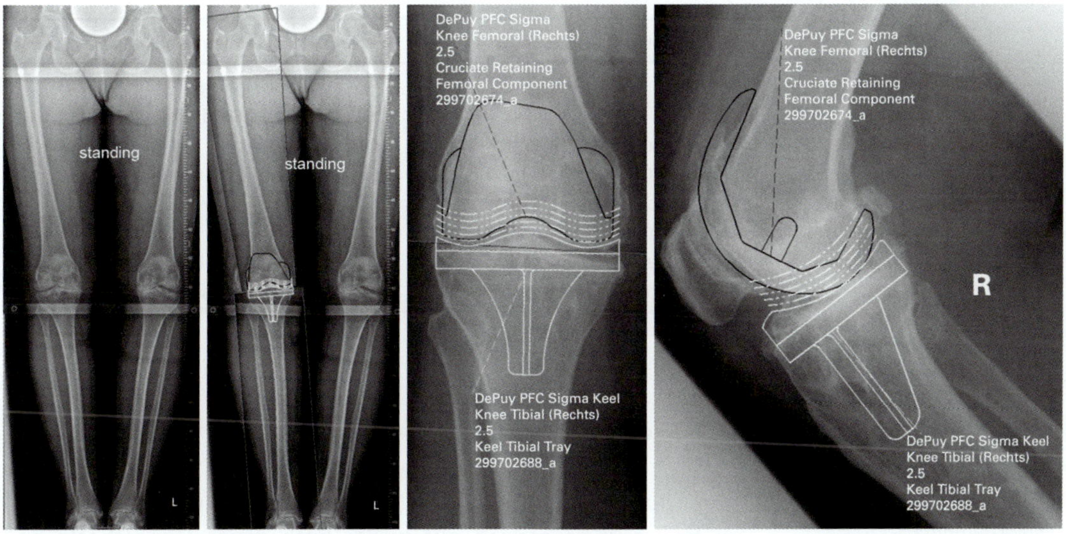

Fig. 3.6: Planning outline with axial correction and size determination of the implant components.

Planning programs for digital imaging and archiving

tion the mediolateral tibial expansion. With the digital imaging and archiving (PACS), planning programs are coming into use (Fig. 3.6). Features of planning can arise as a result of complex situations, for example, in bony defect zones in need of augmentation or distinct deformities with contractures.

3.7.2 Informing Patients

Legally required: discussion, oral or written patient consent to the planned intervention

Standardized information sheet with the possibility of expansion for individual features

Postoperative pain reduction and functional improvement significantly later in knee joint endoprosthetics than in hip endoprosthetics

Legally, the patient should be informed in the case of an elective intervention at least 24 hours preoperatively. Each surgical intervention in accordance with § 229 of the German Criminal Code) represents a physical injury, which has only no legal consequences for the surgeon if there is preoperative discussion and oral or written patient consent to the planned intervention. The use of a standardized information sheet with the relevant possibilities of expansion for individual features has been proven. As well as the execution of the operation and possible alternative therapies, the general and specific surgical risks should be explained to the patient (Table 3.2). Also, the expected time course concerning the postoperative result is of interest to the patient. Here, it should be pointed out that the reduction in pain and improvement in function expected postoperatively is usually slower in comparison to hip endoprosthetics and that the definitive surgical result is evaluable after 6–12 months at the earliest.

Table 3.2: General and specific complications.

General complications	Specific complications
Hematoma	Aseptic loosening
Infection	Axial/rotational deficit
Wound healing impairment	Luxation
Deep vein thrombosis/embolism	Periprosthetic fractures
Intraoperative damage to vessels, nerves, tendons, ligaments, etc.	Limitation of movement
Persistence of the complaint	Difference in leg length
If necessary, another operation	Heterotopic ossifications

3.7.3 Anesthetic Procedures

General anesthesia and spinal/peridural anesthesia possible

The partial and total endoprosthetic replacement of the knee joint can basically be carried out under both general anesthesia and spinal forms of narcosis (spinal/peridural anesthesia). Of vital significance for fast rehabilitation and a good functional surgical result is adequate intra- and postoperative pain therapy, as the endoprosthetic replacement of the knee joint is from experience more painful than that of the hip joint. Because in general anesthesia the perioperative stress response can usually only be controlled by high doses of opiates, spinal or peripheral regional anesthetic procedures (e.g., peridural anesthesia, catheter-assisted nerve/plexus blockade come into use, which can be reused as analgesia in the early postoperative course.

Adequate intra- and postoperative pain therapy important

Endoprosthetic replacement of the knee joint more painful than that of the hip joint

3.8 Perioperative Measures

Perioperative measures

- Blood arrest (used for as short at time as possible during the cementing phase)
- Perioperative antibiotic prophylaxis (single-shot antibiosis – one-off intravenous dose of an antibiotic for short-lasting perioperative antibiotic screen, e.g., with cefuroxime 1.5 g i.v.)
- Donor blood-saving measures (e.g., autotransfusion with drainage blood preparation)
- Intraoperative X-ray image intensifier in special cases
- Thrombosis prophylaxis with low-molecular-weight heparin (LMWH)

3.9 Postoperative Measures

3.9.1 General Postoperative Measures

General postoperative measures

- Investigation of neurovascular status
- General therapeutic measures: cryotherapy, elevation, compression
- Removal of drains 12–24 hours postoperatively
- Special position in extension of the knee joint (heel cushion)
- Thrombosis prophylaxis adjusted for weight and risk (e.g., with low-molecular-weight heparin for 4–6 weeks postoperatively)
- Postoperative X-ray monitoring of the knee joint after removal of the drainage material usually on the 2nd postoperative day, one two planes, tangential patellar X-ray (if required long leg radiograph to analyze the postoperative mechanical leg axis)
- Again providing the patient with in-depth information on the range of movement, load-bearing capacity, and physiotherapeutic after-care
- Individual postoperative physiotherapy, first mobilization can in principle begin on the day of the operation. Depending on

the type of intervention and the individual situation of the patient, physiotherapeutic mobilization and exercise of the joint should be started as early as possible to prevent any possible postoperative complications (thrombosis, pulmonary embolism, movement deficiency). If individual structuring of weight-bearing is required, depending on the implant design and mode of fixation, if necessary, exercise on a motorized splint (CPM)
– Regular check-ups with clinical and if necessary radiological follow-up (e.g., 1 year, 3 years, 5 years, 10 years postoperatively)

3.9.2 Postoperative Pain Therapy

The guarantee of sufficient postoperative pain therapy is not only a legal medical obligation, it is also the fundamental requirement for early mobilization and adequate physiotherapeutic after-care. Postoperative pain is predominantly included in the group of nociceptive pains, with postoperative pain after knee joint interventions often being more pronounced in comparison to hip joint operations. Inadequate pain therapy is a predictive factor for a bad functional result after implantation of a knee joint prosthesis, which also accords vital significance to systematic and quality-assured pain therapy. The objectivization of the postoperative pain level with the aid of visual analog scales (e.g., VAS 0–10, 0 = no pain, 10 = maximum pain imaginable) or numerical rating scales (NRS) should be carried out and documented regularly.

Inadequate pain therapy a predictive factor for a bad functional result

Among the basic therapeutic pain measures are cryotherapy, elevation, and compression if necessary with positioning of the operated extremity in slight flexion to reduce the swelling as well as the release of pain and inflammatory mediators. Early physiotherapeutic mobilization is also conducive to pain relief. Supported by the use of manual lymph drainage to reduce swelling and hematoma, improvement in the complaint can be attained. Pharmacological pain therapy should be carried out in accordance with the three-step concept of the WHO (Fig. 3.7).

Pain therapy:
- Basic therapeutic pain measures
- Early physiotherapeutic mobilization
- Lymph drainage
- Pharmacological pain therapy

Among the specific postoperative analgesic procedures that are being implemented with increasing success is patient-controlled analgesia (PCA), where the control of the intravenous pain therapy (e.g., with piritramide) is left to the patient with the use of programmed pump systems with definable dosage intervals and upper limits. Good patient compliance is vital for this.

Patient-controlled analgesia with use of programmed pump systems

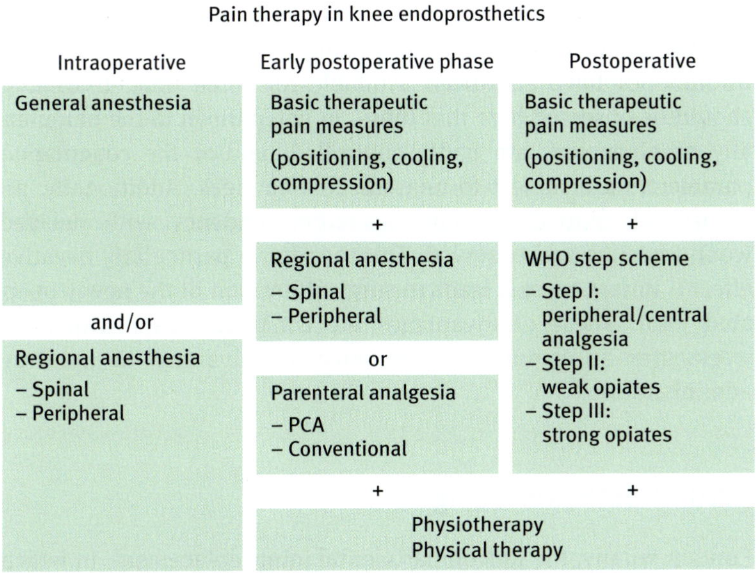

Fig. 3.7: Panesthetic procedures, peri- and postoperative analgesic measures.

Other specific analgesic procedures that are established particularly in the early postoperative phase, are catheter-assisted regional anesthesia procedures such as peridural analgesia or peripheral nerve blockades (e.g., "3-in-1 block": procedure of the peripheral regional anesthesia in which the N. femoralis, N. cutaneous femoris lateralis, and the N. obturatorius are blocked by the placing of a catheter and application of local anesthesia via an inguinal approach to the plexus lumbalis). They are often used intraoperatively and are preferred to isolated systemic opiate therapy on the basis of non-existent sedation and high efficiency at a low risk. Possible undesirable effects like temporary sensory or motoric impairment, however, must be taken into consideration, especially in view of a possible limitation of mobility.

Catheter-assisted regional anesthesia procedures:
- Peridural analgesia
- Peripheral nerve blockades

- No sedation and high efficiency at a low risk

3.9.3 Medical Thrombosis Prophylaxis

According to the guidelines of specialist associations artificial joint replacement operations at the knee joint are high-risk operations, which must accordingly be carried out under medical thrombosis prophylaxis. Thrombosis prophylaxis is commonly conducted using a low-molecular-weight heparin, which is permitted for the high-risk field. The necessity of a medical thrombosis prophylaxis is undisputed, since its duration after a knee prosthesis operation should be six weeks.

Endoprosthetic interventions at the knee joint are among the high-risk operations

Medical thrombosis prophylaxis required

Low-molecular-weight heparins have been proven

Oral antithrombotics have disadvantages

For the medical prophylaxis various low-molecular-weight heparins have been proven to be of value. Orally administered antithrombotics have also been available for some time. Indeed, it should be observed here that these, in comparison to the parenterally administered, are badly controlled, and/or the coagulation parameters are subject to unassessable changes. Additionally, an occasional, extended wound secretion tendency with delayed wound healing was observed. This then has a particularly negative effect if in rare cases it leads to surgical revision of the newly operated joint. These disadvantages are confronted in the first six weeks after an operation by the perceived advantage of oral drug administration.

3.10 Prosthesis Design

Uni-, bi-, and tricompartmentalized joint replacement

Fundamentally, the unicompartmental joint replacement, in which only a femorotibial joint compartment (medial or lateral) is replaced, is distinguished from the bi- (femoral–tibial) and tricompartmental (femorotibial and retropatellar) joint replacement (Fig. 3.8). The unicompartmental replacement of the femoropatellar groove is only rarely carried out in Germany at present and is reserved for a specific spectrum of indications. Furthermore, with

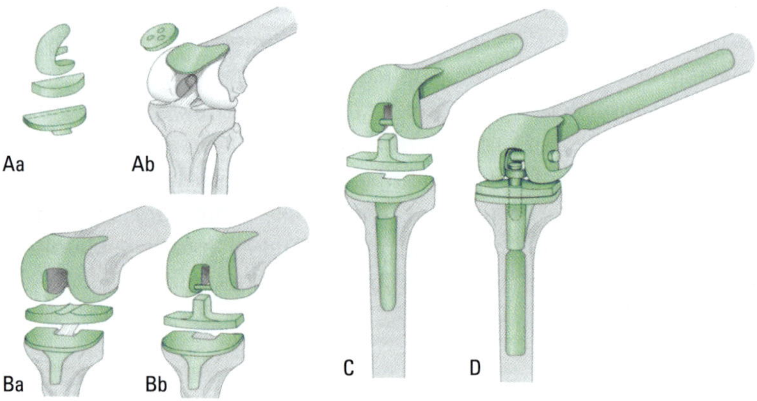

Fig. 3.8: Prosthesis design:.
A Unicompartmental resurfacing, (a) femorotibial/unicondylar, (b) femoropatellar.
B Bicondylar resurfacing, (a) with preservation of the posterior cruciate ligament ("cruciate retaining"), (b) with preservation of the posterior cruciate ligament ("cruciate substituting/posterior stabilized").
C Partly constrained prosthesis ("semi-constrained").
D Axis-guided constrained prosthesis ("constrained, rotating hinge").
(Source: Fraitzl CR et al. Kniegelenk-Arthrose und Arthritis. Orthopädie und Unfallchirurgie up2date 2008;3:155–232).

regard to the stabilizing features of total endoprosthesis unconstrained, partially constrained, and hinged implants are differentiated, which are used independently of the preexisting ligamentous guidance of the joint to be operated on.

Unconstrained, partially constrained, and hinged implants

3.10.1 Unicondylar Joint Replacement (Sled Prosthesis)

The concept of unicondylar joint replacement (Fig. 3.9) was developed for the treatment of isolated medial or lateral joint destruction with intact ligaments and broad physiological axis ratios. Through the continual optimization of the prosthesis design, the implantation instrumentarium, and the surgical technique, as well as through a clearly defined spectrum of indications with precise patient selection, the durability of the current sled prostheses are comparable to that of bicondylar resurfacing.

Unicondylar joint replacement in isolated medial or lateral joint destruction with intact ligaments and physiological axial ratios

Unicompartmental joint replacement versus total endoprosthetic provision

The advantages of a unicompartmental joint replacement versus total endoprosthetic provision have been discussed controversially in the literature since their introduction at the beginning of the 1970s. The unicondylar sled prosthesis is significantly less invasive and guarantees the knee joint function to be as natural as possible through the preservation of all non-damaged structures of the knee joint (especially the cruciate ligaments).

Unicondylar sled prosthesis:
- Less invasive
- Natural knee joint function

Through the possibility of an increasingly used minimally invasive implantation technique in which the prosthesis components can be implanted over a parapatellar mini-arthrotomy without eversion of the patella, less soft-tissue trauma with less intraoperative blood loss compared with the bicondylar resurfacing ensues, which is associated with less peri- and postoperative morbidity. Studies were able to show that intra- and postoperative complications occur less frequently and are less severe. Also, a faster reha-

- Rarer peri- and postoperative complications
- Faster rehabilitation course

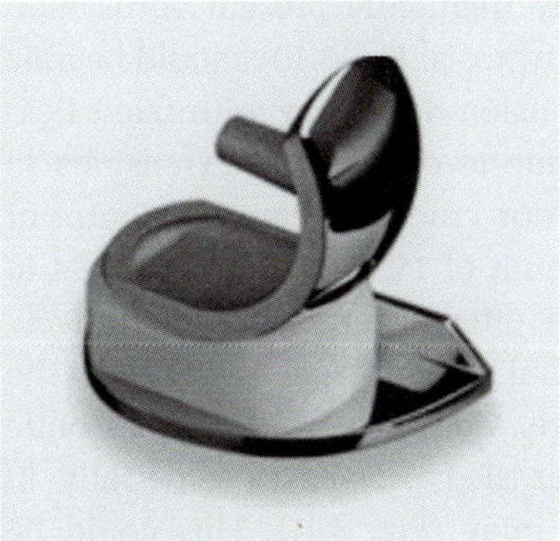

Fig. 3.9: Unicondylar resurfacing (implant, medial sled prosthesis).

bilitation period in comparison to total endoprosthetic joint replacement could be verified.

▸ Technically challenging procedure with corresponding learning curve

A considerable disadvantage of the unicondylar joint replacement lies in the fact that it is a technically challenging and "less forgiving" procedure with a corresponding learning curve. Studies were able to show that surgeons in clinics with a high frequency of operations ("high volume surgery") were able to achieve significantly better results than surgeons who perform the operation only occasionally.

Surgical principle

Surgical principle. Partial endoprosthetic replacement of the medial or lateral knee joint compartment through a femoral metallic sled (sled prosthesis) and a tibial metallic plate with fixed or mobile polyethylene inlay. The operation lasted approximately 60–90 minutes.

Other indications: osteonecrosis, large osteochondral defects

Patient selection and spectrum of indications. Indications for unicondylar joint replacement are purely unicompartmental tibiofemoral joint destruction in patients who display intact ligaments with extensive physiological axial ratios. Here, the entity of anteromedial gonarthrosis constitutes the main indication. Other indications are extensive osteonecrosis (Ahlbäck's disease) or large osteochondral defects that are no longer treatable with conservative or joint-preserving measures.

"One finger sign" for pain localization in anteromedial arthrosis

Medial sled prosthesis. Ideally, the patient with anteromedial arthrosis during clinical questioning about the overriding pain localization presents the so-called "one finger sign", which means that he points to the anteromedial joint space of the affected knee joint with a finger.

Requirements for medial sled prosthesis

In radiologically manifest medial-sided degeneration, the lateral joint compartment in intact meniscus should display completely preserved cartilage thickness, which can be verified by a preserved joint space size in valgus stress radiographs of the knee joint in 20° flexion. The clinically frequently present varus malalignment of the joint (varus gonarthrosis, Fig. 3.10) should be able to be passively corrected; an extension deficiency with fixed flexion contracture, which is often due to osteophytic extensions in the area of insertion of the anterior cruciate ligament "footprint osteophytes," should be a maximum of 15°. Arthrotic changes of the femoropatellar joint, which are often observed intraoperatively in the form of erosions on the medial patellar facet as well as in the area of the medial trochlea femoris, do not represent an absolute contraindication to a unicondylar sled prosthesis, especially in implants with a mobile bearing inlay (Fig. 3.11). This could be

Arthrotic changes in the femoropatellar joint not an absolute contraindication

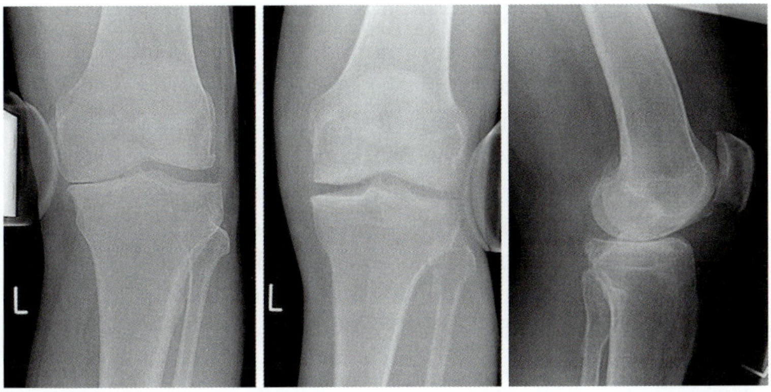

Fig. 3.10: Varus gonarthrosis, varus and valgus stress radiographs, lateral view.

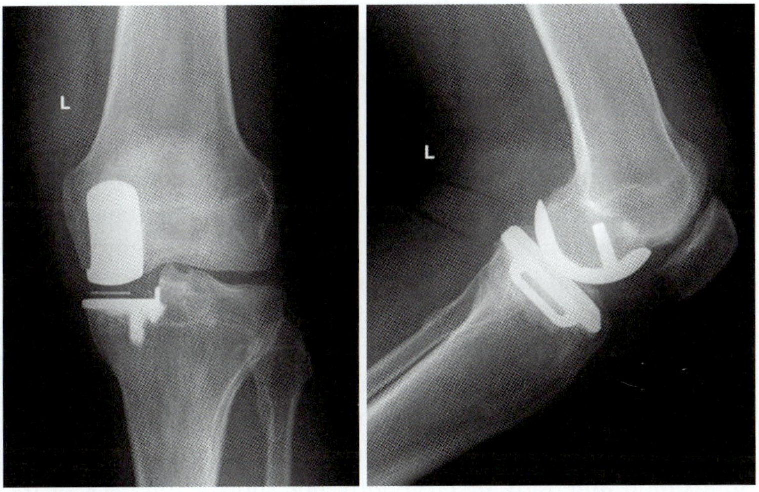

Fig. 3.11: Unicondylar sled prosthesis with mobile bearing inlay, a.p. and lateral views.

shown in several studies and is attributed to a postoperative mechanical unloading of the affected cartilage area (as with the conversion) by the correction of the varus malalignment. Here, attention must be paid to the fact that contrary to total endoprosthetic joint replacement, compensation for the medial signs of wear was the aim and not total correction of the mechanical axis.

Not a complete correction of the mechanical axis, but compensation for medial signs of wear

The aim of unicondylar joint replacement is the physiological reproduction of a knee joint kinematics as far as possible with balanced ligament tension. The anterior and posterior cruciate ligaments must be intact, as stabilization of the knee joint is not guaranteed in the sagittal plane because of the implant.

Aim: reproduction of a physiological knee joint kinematics with balanced ligament tension

Patient age no contraindication

Low morbidity of the unicondylar joint replacement compared with total prosthesis

The patient's age does not represent any contraindication to a sled prosthesis either. The low morbidity of the unicondylar joint replacement on the basis of the low intraoperative soft-tissue trauma and blood loss in minimally invasive implantation is a clear advantage compared with the option of a total prosthesis in older patients. Even in younger patients (50+) a medial sled can be recommended, as the revision rate after an interval of 10 to 15 years is not higher than with alternative total endoprosthetic provision. It can also be shown that the 10-year survival rate in patients in their 50s does not differ significantly from that of older patients (both >90 %). Furthermore, unicondylar replacement offers the advantage that a possible revision is usually surgically relatively simple to design and that revision surgery changing to a bicondylar surface implant shows good results.

Unicondylar replacement: possible revision relatively simple, revision surgery changing to bicondylar surface implant shows good results

Being moderately overweight unproblematic

Being moderately overweight does not have a negative influence on the long-term result.

A quarter of endoprosthetically treated knee joints suitable

If the abovementioned criteria are fulfilled, around every fourth knee that is awaiting endoprosthetic provision is suitable for a medial sled prosthesis.

Precise indication status and adequate preoperative planning essential for success of unicondylar provision

Preoperative planning. A precise indication status combined with adequate preoperative planning is of paramount importance to the success of unicondylar provision. Preoperatively, X-rays of the affected knee joint in two planes as well as varus and valgus stress radiographs should be made. Classically, a loss in the medial-sided joint space is shown on this with classic signs of arthrosis. On the valgus stress radiographs the lateral compartment in relation to the height of the joint space should usually be displayed. On the lateral view the tibia, in comparison to the femur, may neither produce a subluxation anteriorly or posteriorly nor show a roll-back of the tibial plateau with a defect zone reaching posteriorly, as this can be classed as insufficiency of the anterior cruciate ligament and thus a contraindication to unicondylar joint replacement.

Contraindication: insufficiency of the anterior cruciate ligament

Lateral sled prostheses:

- In rare isolated lateral gonarthrosis with intact ligaments
- Only in a few specialized centers
- Surgical technique very challenging

Lateral sled prosthesis. The implantation of lateral sled prostheses (Fig. 3.12) is reserved for the rare isolated lateral gonarthrosis with intact ligaments and is offered in only a few specialized centers. In comparison to medial gonarthrosis, the cartilage defect zone in isolated varus posterolateral gonarthrosis is located posterolaterally. On conventional X-rays in a.p. projection the extent of the chondral destruction cannot therefore be adequately evaluated, which is why a Rosenberg view in 40° flexion should be taken (Fig. 3.13). On the basis of the high mobility of the lateral compartment the surgical technique is also very challenging and requires great precision.

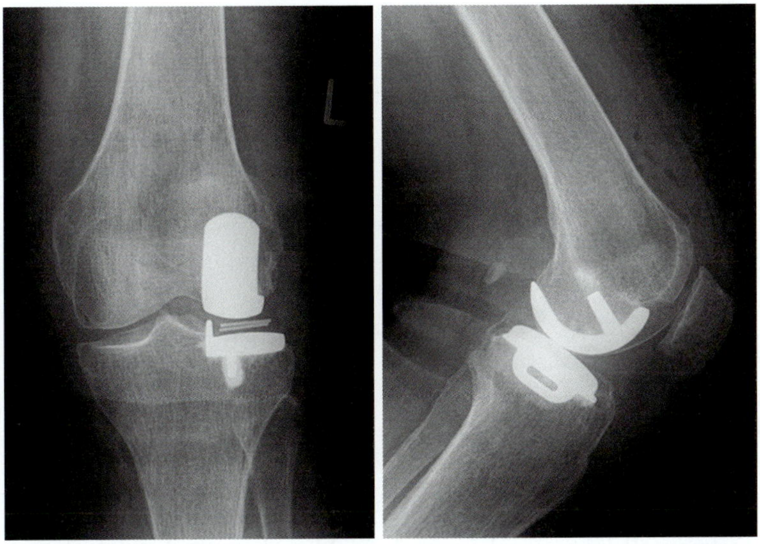

Fig. 3.12: Lateral sled prosthesis, a.p. and lateral.

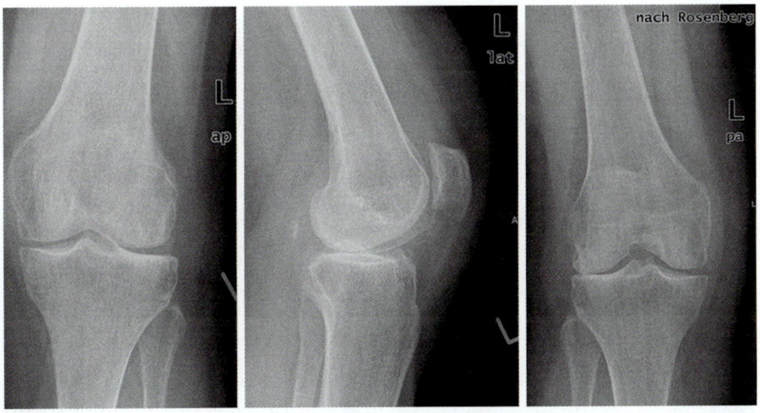

Fig. 3.13: Valgus gonarthrosis, a.p., lateral, p.a., Rosenberg view with complete loss of the lateral joint space in posterolateral defect zone.

3.10.2 Unconstrained Bicondylar Resurfacing

Since the mid-1980s the "unconstrained" resurfacing (Fig. 3.14) has been established as the standard therapy for gonarthrosis with sufficient ligamentous joint control. It enables a rolling-gliding process based on the normal knee function with limited possibility to rotate. In comparison to constrained implants, a significant reduction in the force exerted on the implant fixation is shown.

Unconstrained resurfacing standard therapy for gonarthrosis with adequate ligamentous joint control

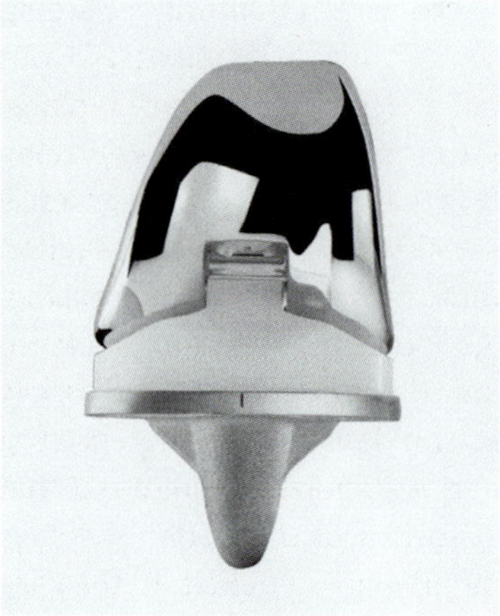

Fig. 3.14: Bicondylar resurfacing (implant).

Surgical principle

Surgical principle. Total endoprosthetic resurfacing (bi- or tricompartmental) by a metal femoral shield and a metal tibial plateau with fixed or mobile polyethylene inlay and the option of retropatellar replacement (polyethylene). The operation lasts around 60–120 minutes.

Indication: advanced pangonarthrosis
Requirements

Patient selection and spectrum of indications. The classic indication for unconstrained resurfacing (Fig. 3.15) is advanced pangonarthrosis. An essential requirement is adequate ligamentous stability through intact collateral ligaments, which guarantee the traction of the prosthesis. The anterior cruciate ligament (ACL) is not required and is resected in the case of most implants. A malalignment of the leg axis in the anterior plane should not be more than 25°. A fixed flexion contracture should not exceed 20°.

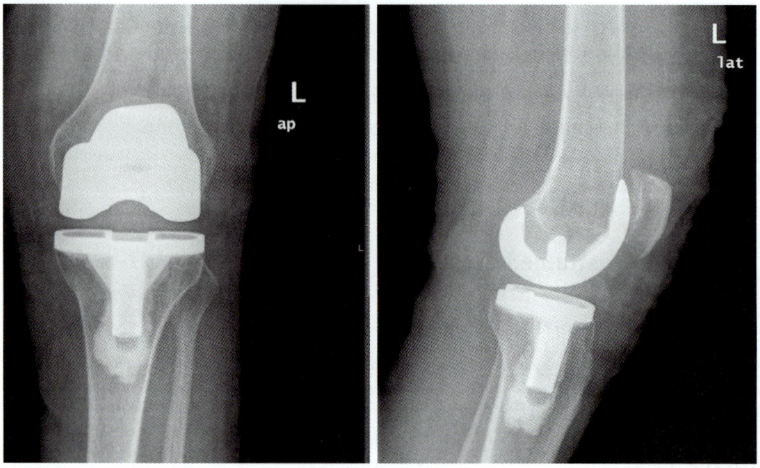

Fig. 3.15: Bicondylar resurfacing, a.p. and lateral.

Cruciate ligament-preserving vs. cruciate ligament-replacing methods. The significance of the posterior cruciate ligament (PCL) for functional results after implantation of a bicondylar surface replacement is a matter for controversial scientific discussion. ACL-replacing implants use specially configured inlays that increase the congruence of the prosthesis components and stabilize the joint in the sagittal plane with a peg in the notch area. Authors who endorse the prosthesis design with presentation of the PCL ("cruciate retaining") refer to the stabilizing and proprioceptive qualities of the PCL as well as low intracondylar bone loss. Surgeons who favor the PCL-replacing implants ("cruciate substituting/posterior stabilized") point out that the PCL, especially in the case of distinct arthrosis, often displays structural damage, with corresponding functional deficit. In the case of fixed valgus arthrosis and flexion contracture in particular, resection of the PCL is often required for correction of the deformity.

Controversial discussion: significance of the posterior cruciate ligament for functional results after implantation of a bicondylar surface replacement

Posterior cruciate ligament with stabilizing and proprioceptive qualities

Fixed valgus gonarthrosis and flexion contractures: resection of the posterior cruciate ligament required for correction of the deformity

Retropatellar replacement. The replacement of the patellar surface is carried out using a polyethylene component that can be cemented directly onto the retropatellar resection surface. The necessity of retropatellar replacement is controversially discussed in the literature. In patients with a well-preserved patellar surface and normal patellar control a retropatellar replacement, according to current studies, can usually be dispensed with. On the other hand, the retropatellar replacement should be carried out in cases of symptomatic retropatellar arthrosis as well as in older patients, femoropatellar dysplasia, and progressively destructive joint diseases (e.g., rheumatoid arthritis).

Controversial discussion: necessity of retropatellar replacement

Mobile vs. fixed bearing. Knee joint and prostheses are divided with regard to bearing into mobile bearing and fixed bearing variants. As opposed to fixed bearing implants in which the polyethylene inlay is fixed to the tibial components, with the mobile bearing prostheses a gliding and/or rotation of the inlay within predetermined limitations is possible. Differentiation is made between the mobile bearing in floating (a.p. translation and rotational movements) and rotating platform (design limited to internal and external rotation) models. Prostheses with mobile bearing surfaces made of polyethylene are offered by almost all prosthesis manufacturers, as, compared with the fixed bearing, they theoretically provide potential advantages. As well as a low amount of wear on the basis of the high contact surface over a large range of motion (dynamic conformity) mobile bearing inlays can compensate for possible rotational defects of the tibial components. As the inlay of the femoral components can adapt dynamically, the physiological roll-glide-rotate movement of the knee joint is better mimicked than with a fixed bearing.

Bearing:
- Floating and rotating platform models
- Low friction
- Compensation for possible rotational defects
- Better mimicking of the physiological roll-glide-rotation of the knee of joint

Disadvantage: subluxation phenomena with soft-tissue impingement

No advantage of mobile compared with fixed glide bearing with regard to durability

A considerable disadvantage of the mobile bearing consists of subluxation phenomena occurring with soft-tissue impingement. Dislocations of the inlay ("spin-out") are also described. No advantages of the mobile as opposed to the fixed bearing, with regard to long-term durability, have yet been documented. Particularly in younger patients under 60 years of age, however, the option of a mobile bearing implant is not contemplated.

Cementless fixation of the femoral shield with good results

In the long run frequent osteolysis in cementless tibial components

Gold standard: cemented implant fixation because of the longest durability and lowest revision rates

Fixation principles. Basically, resurfacing prostheses can be fixed to bone with cement as well as cement-free. Hybrid systems are also available. While the cementless fixation of the femoral shield shows good results in the long run osteolysis occurs more frequently with cementless tibial components than with cemented ones, which among other things is attributed to defective sealing for the prosthesis–bone interface and the associated wear-related osteolysis. In most studies the cemented implant fixation, with the longest durability and lowest revision rates, has proved to be the most reliable method (Swedish Knee Arthroplasty Register). It is therefore still considered to be the gold standard in the fixation of resurfacing prostheses.

3.10.3 Semi-Constrained Prostheses

Partial balancing of ligamentous instabilities in the front and sagittal planes with semi-constrained prostheses

Partially constrained prostheses ("semi-constrained") correspond to the principle of resurfacing and can balance out ligamentous instabilities in the frontal and sagittal planes through design-specific variations of the inlay up to a certain level. A peg in the polyethylene inlay that reinforces the femoral components in an intercondylar box enables stabilization of the knee joint under varus and valgus stress and can thus compensate for this insufficiency of the collateral ligaments.

3.10.4 Hinged Prostheses

Limited reproduction of physiological kinematics of the knee joint by hinged prostheses

Only limited significance in primary endoprosthetics

Hinged prostheses (Figs. 3.16 and 3.17) are modified hinge joints, which can reproduce the physiological kinematics of the knee joints in only a limited way. Since the 1970s good results have been achieved with them in the primary endoprosthetics provision for gonarthrosis; however, they still only have a limited significance owing to the very good long-term results of resurfacing in primary endoprosthetics.

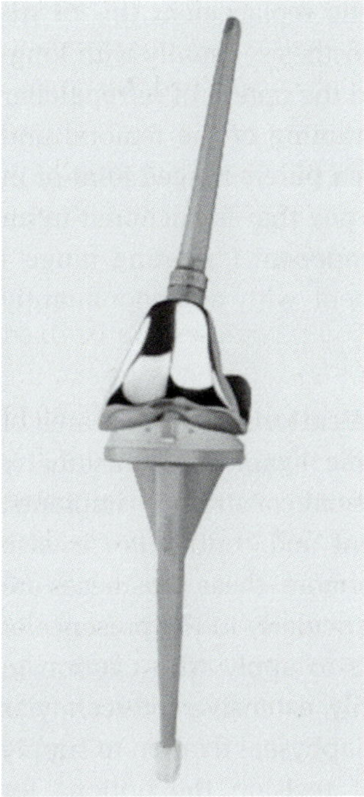

Fig. 3.16: Hinged prosthesis (implant).

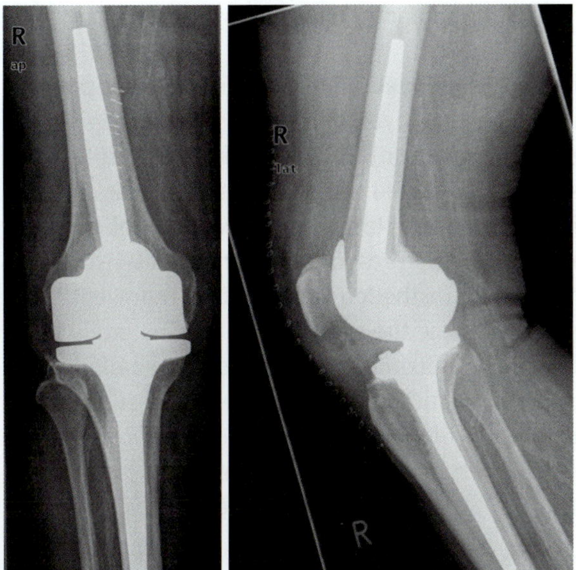

Fig. 3.17: Hinged prosthesis, a.p. and lateral.

Surgical principle

Surgical principle. Total endoprosthetic replacement (bi- or tricompartmental) by a modified hinge prosthesis, usually with long-stemmed tibial and femoral fixation and the option of retropatellar replacement (polyethylene). The constraining of the femoral and tibial components takes place either via a purely hinged joint or in the case of newer implants via a tibial peg that is anchored in an intercondylar space of the femoral component ("rotating hinge") and enables limited rotational movement with a predominantly condylar transfer of force.

Indications:
- Gonarthrosis with chronic ligamentous instability
- Compensation for marked malalignment and contracture
- Revision endoprosthetics, especially in the presence of osseous defect zones

Limited removal options in the case of revision

Patient selection and spectrum of indications. The main area of application is gonarthrosis with chronic ligamentous instability that cannot be compensated for by semi-constrained implants. Compensation for marked malalignment and contracture is also possible with hinged prostheses. Furthermore, these prostheses are applied in revision endoprosthetics, particularly in the presence of osseous defect zones. The indication is to apply with caution in young patients owing to the necessarily extensive intercondylar bone resection and the long-stemmed diaphyseal fixation to supply with caution, because in the case of revision the options for removal are limited.

3.10.5 Modular Revision Implants/Tumor Prostheses

Modular implants and individually manufactured special prostheses in revision endoprosthetics and oncological orthopedics

Great challenge for surgeon and materials used

Long-term results of modular prostheses significantly worse

Modular implants and individually manufactured special prostheses ("custom made") are employed in both revision endoprosthetics and oncological orthopedics (Fig. 3.18). Osseous defect situations, which arise in the treatment of neoplasias as well as complex revision settings, can be treated through the development of modular implants that increasingly preserve the extremities ("limb salvage surgery"). The endoprosthetic reconstruction represents here however a great challenge for the surgeon and the materials used. Because of the complicated fixation, which should usually be carried out diaphyseally, and the complicated reconstruction of the joint biomechanics with high mechanical demands on the implants, the long-term results of modular prostheses are significantly worse than those of primary knee joint endoprostheses.

3.10.6 Patellofemoral Prostheses

Unicompartmental replacement of the femoropatellar joint in specialized centers

The endoprosthetic unicompartmental replacement of the femoropatellar joint is carried out in only a few specialized centers in Germany.

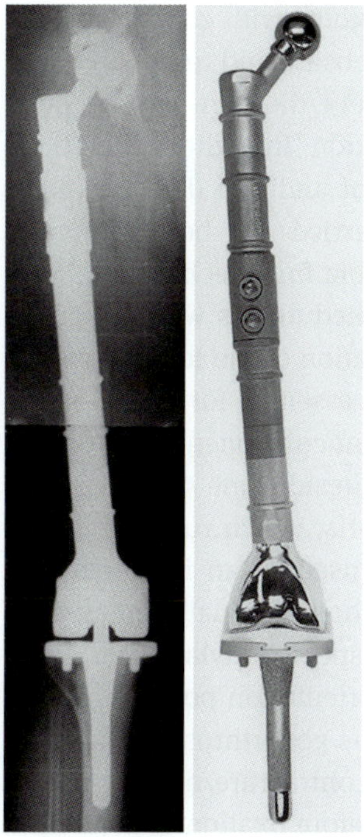

Fig. 3.18: Total femoral replacement in a 20-year-old patient who had undergone multiple previous operations after resection of a Ewing sarcoma with an infectious course.

Surgical principle. Resurfacing of the femoral bearing (trochlea) by a metal shield with replacement of the posterior surface of the patella with a polyethylene component.

Surgical principle

Patient selection and spectrum of indications. An indication for a patellofemoral arthroplasty is the isolated symptomatic retropatellar arthrosis, which is observed in up to 10 % of patients with gonarthrosis. Requirements are regular femoropatellar alignment as well as a joint stabilized by ligaments. An advantage of this method in comparison to total endoprosthetic replacement is the low amount of bone matter lost, with preservation of the natural knee joint kinematics. While the first results of the patellofemoral prostheses demonstrate a high failure rate of up to 50 % after eight years, the middle term results of current studies, with revision-free durability of over 95 % after five years, are promising. A considerable problem, however, is high rate of radiologically manifest arthrosis progression (up to 25 %) with the spread of the degenerative changes to the tibiofemoral compartment.

Indication: isolated, symptomatic retropatellar arthrosis

Advantage: loss of a smaller amount of bone substance with preservation of the natural knee joint kinematics

Problem: high arthrosis progression rate with spread of the degenerative changes to the tibiofemoral compartment

3.11 Surgical Technique

The routine approach to implantation of a knee joint total endoprosthesis is made via a ventral-sided straight skin incision with a con-

Routine approach

secutive medial-sided parapatellar arthrotomy with conservation of the patellar ligament. After soft-tissue exposure and resection of the menisci and the anterior cruciate ligament the joint can be positioned with eversion of the patella in flexion. In addition, the bone resections are conducted after adjustment and size determination, thus, the initial preparation can be carried out both femorally ("femur first" technique) and tibially ("tibia first" technique). Here, intra- and extramedullary alignment procedures as well as special saw blocks can be applied with consideration of the femoral valgus angle. The exact determination of ratio is essential for a good surgical result. For the alignment of the implant components anatomical landmarks (posterior condylar plane, Whiteside Line = anteroposterior line in the area of the trochlea femoris, which runs vertical to the transepidcondylar axis and can be used as an intraoperative anatomical landmark for orientation in the rotational alignment of the femoral implant components; transpepicondylar axis, tibial tuberosity, tibial ridge, etc. are used as orientation points.

Initial preparation femoral ("femur first" techniques) or tibial ("tibia first" technique)

Exact rotation determination essential for good surgical result

In osseous matter defects (e.g., valgus gonarthrosis with hypoplastic lateral condyles, osteonecrosis, contracture/malalignment) the risk of malpositioning is increased. Before fixation of the definitive implants residual osteophytes are removed and test components are positioned for the evaluation of range of motion and joint stability. The aim is a joint stabilized by ligaments with even, symmetrical extension and flexion spaces. If adequate soft-tissue balance is achieved, the original implants are brought to the surgical site after careful washing (e.g., jet lavage, especially with cemented fixation).

High risk of malpositioning in osseous matter defects

Aim: joint stabilized by ligaments with even symmetrical extension and flexion spaces

3.11.1 Alternative Surgical Approaches

MIS. In endoprosthetics of the knee joint minimally invasive surgical methods (MIS) are also increasingly used. The exposure of the surgical site is carried out in a minimized manner as the midvastus or subvastus approach without eversion of the patella.

Increasing minimally invasive surgical methods

Overview limited in comparison to the conventional procedure

In a minimally invasive procedure lower morbidity compared with the conventional implantation is assumed owing to the lower intraoperative soft-tissue trauma and blood loss. Furthermore, some comparative studies show accelerated rehabilitation in the first postoperative weeks, thus it is noticeable that from the 6th postoperative week no statistically significant advantage over conventional implantation techniques could be proven.

Minimally invasive procedures:
- Low morbidity
- Accelerated rehabilitation in the first postoperative weeks

The real positive effect of the present minimally invasive procedures is not currently evaluable owing to the low number of randomized and controlled studies and the lack of long-term results.

Evidence-based assessment not possible (fewer studies, long-term results lacking)

Also, the term minimally invasive is inadequately defined, thus, a final evidence-based assessment of less invasive surgical techniques is still to come.

Tibia first vs. femur first. The tibia-first technique is a soft-tissue-oriented surgical method that is often applied in connection with a minimally invasive approach. After resection of the tibial plateau and the distal femur in extension a balanced extension gap is aimed for through soft-tissue release. Soft-tissue balancing of the extension gap occurs with the aid of spacers. In addition, the rotational alignment of the femoral components is referred to by means of the soft-tissue tension of the functional flexion gap. The removal of the posterior condyle osteophytes is more difficult with use of this method.

Tibia-first technique:
- Soft tissue oriented surgical method, usually minimally invasive approach
- Rotational alignment of the femoral components with the aid of soft-tissue tension of the function flexion gap

In traditional femur-first technique the alignment of the implant's components occurs with the aid of bony anatomical landmarks.

Femur-first technique: component alignment with the aid of bony anatomical landmarks

Navigation. In contrast to the conventional referencing methods of implant alignment, with the assistance of the instrumentarium, in navigational knee joint endoprosthetics the resection planes are ascertained with computerized support (CAS: computer assisted surgery). After appropriate exposure of the joint, special markers (trackers) are attached to particular landmarks which help the computer system to determine the resection planes. Furthermore, in the newer systems computer-supported soft-tissue balancing with evaluation of ligamentous tension over the whole range of motion of the knee joint is also available. The main aim of the use of navigation systems is to optimize the precision of the implantation. Several studies were able to show that a connection exists between axially precise implantation and the durability of the prosthesis, thus, from a discrepancy of more than 3° from the neutral leg axis, it is assumed that there will be an increase in polyethylene wear. In Germany significantly less than 20 % of all knee joint implants are carried out with navigation, as the considerable disadvantages of navigational implantation lie in an extended operation time and greater exposure of the surgical site.

In navigational knee endoprosthetics computer-assisted determination of the resection planes

Computer-assisted soft-tissue balancing with evaluation of the ligamentous tension over the whole range of motion of the knee joint
Aim: optimization of the precision of the implantation

Disadvantages:
- Extended operating time
- Greater exposure of the surgical site

A further development in navigation, meanwhile, consists in the manufacture of custom-made guiding instruments, which are deployed by the surgeon during the operation at the surgical site and enable resection of the bone that has been preplanned on the computer. For this purpose, several weeks before the operation a CT or MRT of the whole leg is carried out, with the aid of which the surgeon plans the operation in advance on the computer and determines both the axial alignment and the prosthesis size.

Further development of navigation: manufacture of custom-made guiding instruments

Soft-tissue situation and/or ligamentous tension are disregarded

Finally, the individual molds are manufactured that are used for the operation. Both in the navigation and in the custom-made guiding instruments the soft-tissue situation and/or the ligamentous tension are disregarded, which is of considerable significance for the balancing of the knee joint.

Conventional continuation of the operation possible at any time

At any time during a navigation or individualized operation the surgeon is in a position to continue the operation in the conventional manner.

Navigation, individualized endoprosthetics only for experienced surgeons

Navigation and individualized endoprosthetics should only be applied by experienced surgeons, as only the experienced is "master of the system" at any time and can judge whether the operation is proceeding correctly. This means that these technical aids are no substitution for the surgeon's lack of experience.

3.12 Complications

General and specialized complications

Possible complications in endoprosthetics of the knee joint can be divided into general and specialized complications. Because of the increasing number of implantations and the demographic development, the absolute number of complications requiring revision is also rising. The revision rate in the first two postoperative years after primary implantation lies at around 3 %. The most common causes of revisions are polyethylene wear/aseptic loosening, instability, and infections. Factors that increase the risk of a complication requiring revision are male gender, age under 55 years at the time of the operation, being overweight, and existing comorbidities

Most common causes of revisions: polyethylene friction/aseptic loosening, instability, infections

Risk factors

3.12.1 General Complications

- Thrombosis/embolism
- Postoperative hematoma
- Vascular and axonal injury
- Wound healing disorders

3.12.2 Specialized Complications

Increased polyethylene wear owing to the complex geometry of the knee joint

Wear and aseptic loosening. Polyethylene wear and consequent osteolysis constitute a crucial factor that influences the long-term survival of knee joint endoprosthesis. In contrast to the highly congruent articulation of hip joint endoprostheses, in knee joint implants, owing to the complex geometry of the knee joint, increased polyethylene wear with large polyethylene particles and delamination occurs and leads to wear-induced aseptic loosening and to instability, which are associated with wear-induced loss of matter. The extent of the wear is dependent upon the patient's level of activity, the quality of the polyethylene as well as upon the implant design.

Extent of the wear dependent upon patient activity, polyethylene quality, implant design

Anterior knee pain/patellofemoral pain. Anterior knee pain after endoprosthetic interventions at the knee joint occur in up to 15 % of patients in various forms. In this context, possible rotational faults, especially malpositioning of the femoral components in internal rotation with patella maltracking, are discussed. The necessity for a general retropatellar replacement is also the subject of scientific controversy. In spite of comprehensive diagnostic possibilities for the precise determination of the positioning of the implant (rotational CT), the cause of anterior knee pain frequently remains unclear.

Anterior knee pain after endoprosthetic interventions at the knee joint in up to 15 % of patients

Cause often unclear

Motion deficit/arthrofibrosis. Postoperative motion limitations with functional deficit are facilitated by various factors. Preoperatively, an existing motion limitation and previous operations constitute a negative predictive factor. Intraoperative malpositioning, inadequate soft-tissue balancing, or insufficient removal of dorsal osteophytes also limit the scope of movement. Postoperatively, insufficient analgesia and infections can facilitate a functional deficit. The preventive use of CPM splints ("continuous passive motion") is recommended in a protracted postoperative course with regard to range of motion. Therapeutic options in persistent motion limitation are closed narcosis mobilization and/or open revision and arthrolysis of the joint with consequent physiotherapy under adequate analgesia, for example, through the use of local anesthetic administered by catheter.

Postoperative motion limitations with functional deficit
Preoperative risk factors

Postoperative risk factors

Therapeutic options

Infection. As well as the classic systemic (fever, shivering) and local signs of infection (flushing, swelling, hyperthermia), persistent wound secretion and prolonged painful motion limitation of the operated joint are also serious signs of infection. According to the timing, early infection (up to the fourth postoperative week) is differentiated from late infection (after the fourth postoperative week). Depending on the severity of the infection, with an early infection, an initial implant-preserving procedure with surgical revision, debridement, thorough rinsing, and a change of inlay with the consequent appropriate antibiotics can be considered. A late infection requires in most cases explantation of the prosthesis with placing of an interpositional space preserver (spacer) made of cement containing antibiotics. In a two-stage revision procedure,

Late infection: usually explantation of the prosthesis and prosthesis revision (two-stage)

the prosthesis reimplantation can take place when there is normalization of the laboratory inflammatory parameters, aseptic aspiration, and non-inflammatory symptoms. The interval of spacer attachment should be at least 6–8 weeks.

One-stage revision in selected cases

In the case of a known configuration of germs in selected individual cases a one-stage revision procedure is possible. Here, the installation and removal of the infected knee prosthesis can be carried out during one operation.

Antibiotic-impregnated bone cement for revision operation

Generally, in infection-induced revision surgery bone cement impregnated with antibiotics is used; according to its antibiogram other specifically effective antibiotics can be admixed.

Risk of infection in primary implantations is around 1–2 %

Increased risk of infection with revisions, particular co-morbidities

The average risk of a prosthesis infection is around 1–2 % in primary implantations; from specialized centers with a high volume of operations the infection rates are quoted as being less than 1 %. If revision scenarios, particular co-morbidities (e.g., diabetes mellitus, rheumatoid arthritis, obesity), and immunosuppression (steroids) are present, a high risk of infection exists, about which the patient should be informed within the scope of the consent to surgery.

Tear of the extensor mechanism by forced flexion and eversion attempts of the patella without adequate soft-tissue mobilization

Increased risk in patients who have undergone several previous operations, patella baja

Injuries to the extensor mechanism. Forced attempts at flexion and eversion of the patella without adequate soft-tissue mobilization can cause a tear of the extensor mechanism, which frequently gives rise to considerable functional limitation. In particular, in patients who have undergone several previous operations and have pronounced scarring, and in cases of patella baja, there is an increased risk, thus, intraoperative safeguarding of the extensor mechanism is applied. Replacement of the extensor mechanism is occasionally required in the case of insufficient joint exposure (tuberosity osteotomy). Tears of the patellar ligament and the quadriceps tendon can be re-fixed transosseously.

Complication: intraoperative injuries to the collateral ligaments, especially the lateral ligament

Indication: persistent joint opening in stability testing after insertion of the sample components

Ligamentous instability. Intraoperative injuries to the collateral ligaments, especially the lateral ligament, represent a formidable complication and manifest through persistent joint opening in stability testing after insertion of the sample components. Causes can be inadequate soft-tissue protection owing to absent or incorrectly positioned soft tissue retractors in the preparation of the femur and/or tibia or inaccurate meniscal resection. A surgical reconstruction can be considered in the injury of collateral ligaments (transosseous refixation, interligamentous suture), but requires a consistent and protracted follow-up with an orthosis. If a stable enough ligamentous reconstruction is not possible, a change of procedure to a semi-constrained or hinged implant must be performed.

Luxation of the patella. Postoperative patellar luxation or subluxation is facilitated by valgus malalignments, patellar dysplasia, and patella alta. If a dysplastic or hypoplastic posterior patellar surface appears intraoperatively, a retropatellar replacement should be carried out. Malpositioning of the implant components in terms of an internal rotation position of the femoral shield or the tibial plateau also contributes to a patellar instability with luxation tendency. In the case of persistent instability in spite of regular implant positioning accompanying soft-tissue procedures (e.g., "lateral release", medial capsular plication) can improve the guidance of the patella. In cases of more persistent patellar subluxation or luxation (maltracking) patella posterior resurfacing with appropriate positioning of the polyethylene posterior surface may also be necessary.

Postoperative patellar luxation or subluxation by valgus malalignment, patellar dysplasia, patella alta

Further causes: malpositioning of the implant components

Patellar maltracking may also occur secondarily and not become symptomatic until years after the prosthesis operation. Here, a secondarily implanted posterior surface replacement, perhaps in combination with a lateral release, is productive.

Patellar maltracking also secondary

Periprosthetic fractures. Periprosthetic fractures can occur both intra- and postoperatively. The predominantly surgical treatment of them is technically challenging and is afflicted with a high complication rate. The incidence lies at around 1%. There is an elevated danger of fracture in patients with osteoporotic bones, and in the malpositioning of the prosthesis components alike. Other risk factors are long-stemmed implants, cementless fixation, and the revision setting. Prognostically significant are the early identification of an intraoperative fracture and the choice of an adequate provision strategy. Aims of the treatment of periprosthetic fractures are the exact repositioning and stable fixation of the fracture as well as the reproduction of an adequate extensor mechanism. Also, early mobilization of the patient is aimed for, to prevent further complications.

Periprosthetic fractures: intra- or postoperative

Surgical therapy technically challenging, high complication rate

Incidence: around 1%

Risk factors

Early identification, adequate provision strategy prognostically significant

Treatment goals

With the correct surgical technique, intraoperative fractures seldom occur and come about predominantly because of blows to the implant components and inadequate stability-impairing saw-cutting. In the case of isolated bone chips an osteosynthetic provision is usually sufficient, whereas in fractures in the condylar or stem area an implant with primary stable fixation is often only possible with a long-stemmed revision implant with simultaneous osteosynthesis.

Intraoperative fractures seldom with correct surgical technique

Treatment

Excessive thinning of the patella in the preparation of the retropatellar joint surface can lead to fractures of the patella. Depending on the type of fracture, various osteosynthesis procedures are used.

Patellar fractures through excessive thinning of the patella

Postoperative fractures in the case of enclosed implants rare

Mechanism of injury

Postoperative periprosthetic fractures in the case of enclosed implants are an unusual complication. The main location is the supracondylar region; tibial and patellar periprosthetic fractures are rarely described. The mechanism of injury is a minor trauma in the case of a fall onto the knee joint; more rarely, high-speed trauma, e.g., in traffic accidents, comes into consideration.

Heterotopic ossification after knee prosthesis implantation rare

Primary prevention: postoperative administration of NSAR

Recurrence prevention: pre- and/or postoperative radiotherapy

Heterotopic ossifications. The occurrence of heterotopic ossifications is considerably less frequently observed than after hip endoprosthetic interventions. However, they can lead to pronounced limitations of movement, that make a surgical revision necessary. Predilection sites are the extensor mechanism and the area of the ventral femur. The postoperative administration of *non-steroidal anti-rheumatics is suitable for primary prevention; the recurrence prevention can be carried out with pre- and/or postoperative radiotherapy.*

3.13 Rehabilitation

Postoperative rehabilitation:
- After-care during the inpatient stay
- Early rehabilitation in rehab clinic or ambulant
- Ambulant late rehab, under care of practicing consultant

Aim: adequate mobility; good, pain-free knee joint function

Postoperative rehabilitation after endoprosthetic interventions at the knee joint includes, in addition to the early after-care within the scope of the postoperative inpatient stay, which lasts around 5–14 days depending on the type of intervention and the individual patient situation, an early rehabilitation period (follow-up treatment in a rehab clinic or ambulant rehab measures, duration approximately 2–3 weeks) and an additional ambulant late rehabilitation period under the care of the practicing consultant. The aim of rehabilitation is to regain adequate mobility and good, pain-free knee joint function in order to ensure reintegration of the patient into their social environment (family, work, leisure, sport) with an improved quality of life.

3.14 Outlook

Endoprosthetic replacement of the knee joint established methods with good long-term results

Continuously increasing numbers of primary implantations and revisions

The endoprosthetic replacement of the knee joint is an established method with good long-term results for implant survival rates and patient satisfaction. Owing to the demographic development and patients' increasing requirement for activity into old age, continuously rising numbers of primary implantations and revisions are anticipated. The basic requirements for a good surgical result are the consideration of patient's individual anatomical and biomechanical factors and the right choice of implant. A precise surgical technique with correct axial alignment and symmetrical balancing of soft-tissue as well as adequate postoperative after-care with sufficient analgesia are also of great importance. Because the causes of failure of knee prostheses are diverse and depend on the complex connections among patient-, implant-, and surgery-related factors, further improvement in the materials used and in surgical techniques is expected. In particular, the field of navigational and minimally invasive methods must hold its own in the face of the good long-term results of proven procedures.

Further improvement in the materials used and in the surgical techniques is expected

References

Ackroyd CE, Newman JH, Evans R, Eldridge JD, Joslin CC. The Avon patellofemoral arthroplasty: Five-year survivorship and functional results. J Bone Joint Surg Br 2007;89-B:310–5.

Aldinger PR, Clarius M, Murray DW, Goodfellow JW, Breusch SJ. Medial unicompartimental knee replacement using the "Oxford Uni" meniscal bearing knee. Orthopäde 2004;33:1277–83.

Buckwalter JA, Saltzman C, Brown T. The impact of osteoarthritis: Implications for research. Clin Orthop Relat Res 2004;45(427 Suppl):6–15.

Buechel FF Sr. Long-term followup after mobile-bearing total knee replacement. Clin Orthop Relat Res 2002;404:40–50.

Burnett RS, Haydon CM, Rorabeck CH, Bourne RB. Patella resurfacing versus nonresurfacing in total knee arthroplasty. Clin Orthop Relat Res 2004;428:12–25.

Callaghan JJ. Mobile-bearing knee replacement: clinical results. A review of the literature. Clin Orthop Relat Res 2001;392:221–5.

Consensus statement on total knee replacement des NIH, 2003, http://consensus. nih.gov/2003/2003TotalKneeReplacement117PDF.pdf.

Duncan RC, Hay EM, Sklatvala J, Croft PR. Prevalence of radiographic osteoarthritis it all depends on your point of view. Rheumatology 2006;45:757–60.

Heisel C, Kinkel S, Bernd L, Ewerbeck V. Megaprostheses for the treatment of malignant bone tumours of the lower limbs. International Orthopaedics 2006;30:452–7.

Lonner JH. Patellofemoral arthroplasty. J Am Acad Orthop Surg 2007; 15(8):495–506.

Mihalko WM, Boachie-Adje Yi, Spang JT, Fulkerson JP, Arendt EA, Saleh KJ. Controversies and techniques in the surgical management of patellofemoral arthritis. J Bone Joint Surg Am 2007;89:2788–802.

Scott RD. Total knee arthroplasy. München: Elsevier, 2005.

Seyler TM, Marker DR, Bhave A, Plate JF, Marulanda GA, Bonutti PM, Delanois RE, Mont MA. Functional problems and arthrofibrosis following total knee arthroplasty. J Bone Joint Surg Am 2007;89(Suppl 3):59–69.

Sharkey PF, Hozack WJ, Rothman RH, Shastri S, Jacoby SM. Why are total knee arthroplasties failing today? Clin Orthop Relat Res 2002;404:7–13.

Su ET, Hargovind D, Di Cesare PE. Periprosthetic femoral fractures above total knee replacement. J Am Acad Orthop Surg 2004;12:12–20.

Wagner KJ, Kochs EF, Krautheim V, Gerdesmeyer L. Perioperative pain therapy for knee endoprosthetics. Orthopäde 2006;35:153–61.

S. Lieske, K. Schenk, M. John, H.W. Neumann

4 Ankle Endoprosthetics

4.1 Introduction

For many decades the stiffening of the ankle was the gold standard in advanced arthrosis of the upper ankle. This particularly affected accident-related arthrosis. The "solution" for the large group of patients who suffer from chronic polyarthritis (rheumatoid arthritis) turned out to be less favorable. For them severe changes are present in the forefoot at the same time; thus, a stiffened ankle subsequently represents quite a considerable extra load on the forefoot and significantly worsens the situation.

Stiffening of the ankles long the gold standard in advanced, accident-related arthrosis of the upper ankle

Problem: patients with chronic polyarthritis

On the other hand, profound osteoporosis near the joint exists in these patients while, for example, patients with post-traumatic arthrosis display osteosclerosis near the joint. Patients with chronic polyarthritis are also burdened by the fact that the adjacent joints (knee joint, the talonavicular joint, and the lower ankle) are often particularly affected and sometimes tend to stiffen.

Posttraumatic arthrosis: osteosclerosis close to the joint

Chronic polyarthritis: osteoporosis close to the joint

Adjacent joints often co-affected

In the last few years, with primary varus and valgus arthrosis of the upper ankle, another group of patients has emerged (estimated frequency 10/1). This disease occurs particularly frequently in patients past 60 years of age, almost always affects both ankles, and leads to severe foot deformities, with excessive loading of the outside edge of the foot (varus arthrosis) or severe flat feet (valgus arthrosis).

Often in patients >60 years: primary varus and valgus arthrosis of the upper ankle

Clinical results after ankle arthrodesis, which are remarkable, face the difficulties mentioned at the beginning that accompany stiffening of the upper ankle. After isolated stiffening of the upper ankles the adjacent joints are often have very good mobility, if they themselves do not show advanced arthrosis at the time of the operation. This is why only slightly worse results in movement appear in patients who have undergone ankle arthrodesis than in patients who have had endoprosthetic implantation. At the same time, it should also be considered that a substantially stiff upper ankle may only gain 10–15° of movement with insertion of an endoprosthesis, a range of motion, that, after abatement of the pain, can also be achieved to a similar extent by stiffening of the ankle. Consequently, the previous approach, waiting as long as possible for the time of the insertion of an endoprosthesis and putting up with a relative stiffening of the joint, is no longer effective today. The worse the movement is at the time of the operation the worse the functional outcome. This also applies for stiffening of the upper ankle.

Good clinical results after ankle arthrodesis

After ankle arthrodesis barely worse results with regard to movement than after endoprosthesis implantation

Substantial stiff upper ankle through endoprosthesis implantation with movement of 10–15°

Functional outcome dependent on movement at the time of the operation

Introductory process of a surgical procedure at the upper joint very complicated

Results dependent on surgical experience of the surgeon

Secondary removal of the prosthesis and transfer to arthrodesis possible

While the fear of "stiffening" of the ankles – often irrational – has brought us 800 patients for surgery over the past ten years, such an introductory phase of a surgical procedure on the upper ankle is indeed very complicated. There exists among colleagues a very critical attitude because the disease frequency is very low and therefore most clinics only have a very low one-digit number of patients at their disposal. Often implants are also revised, although it has been shown in the last few years that the results are less dependent on the type of prosthesis and much more reliant on the surgical experience of the surgeon.

Contrary to some critical comments, we are convinced of the triumph that is endoprosthetics and know that even if a pain-free and well-moving ankle is not achieved, the secondary removal of the prosthesis and a transfer to an arthrodesis of the upper, partly in combination with the lower, joint is possible.

4.2 History

1973 the first ankle prosthesis

Pain reduction at the forefront

In 1973 for the first time an ankle endoprosthesis was implanted by G. Lord and J.H. Marotte. With the materials of the time stable fixation of the implant was only just possible. Indeed, good primary stability was achieved with cemented implantation, but after only a short duration the loosening and revision rates increased drastically. Then as now pain reduction was at the forefront. As these were similarly achieved with arthrodesis and were able to come up with lower complication rates, these became prevalent for a long time and were regarded to be the gold standard. Owing to early failure ankle endoprosthetics were initially regarded as an experimental procedure and moved into the background for many years.

Today, mostly three-component endoprosthesis with cementless fixation

Today's implants are in most cases three-component endoprostheses and are fixed without cement. This offers the advantage that the unconstrained components offer free movement in all planes. Thus, they respect the biomechanical conditions distinctly more than the previous models and attempt to preserve the natural flow of movement in the ankle complex. The first models with this design approach were developed by Buechel, Pappas as well as Kofoed.

Less malalignment and intraoperative fractures through improved range of instruments

An improved range of instruments also plays a large part in the growing success, which makes available to surgically active colleagues systems that minimize the possibility of malalignment and intraoperative fractures.

Another important point is the condition of the surface. The introduction of coating with hydroxyapatite and of porous surfaces guarantees better osseointegration and certainly has a great many better results. Furthermore, modern press-fit procedures increase primary stability. Whichever method will ultimately win through will be shown by the result of the next few years.

Better results owing to coating with hydroxy-apatite, use of porous surfaces, press-fit method

In spite of the increasing promising results the endoprosthetic treatment of the upper ankle has with established colleagues an absurdly bad reputation.

4.3 Implants

The development of suitable implant s for the upper ankle was very difficult to shape at the beginning. In comparison to hip and knee joints the disparately difficult anatomical/biomechanical conditions must be taken into consideration. The joint is comparatively small, has a bone contact surface of only 0.25 m^2 and bears loads that can exceed five times the body weight. The higher the grade of constraint of the prosthesis components (constrained, semiconstrained, unconstrained), the stronger the torque and compressive force that occur. Also, especially in unconstrained three-component models, the ligamentous situation must gain interest, as the control is no longer given owing to the congruent articular surfaces after endoprosthesis implantation.

Development of suitable implants for the upper ankle difficult

Difficult anatomical/bio-mechanical conditions in the ankle

Consideration of all models of ankle endoprosthetics would go beyond the scope of this chapter. In fact, an overview of the current systems that are used in most clinics will be given (Tab. 4.1). Furthermore, for each prosthesis presented, a radiological example will be shown, so that the identification in daily routine is easily accomplished.

Overview of current systems of ankle endoprosthetics

Table 4.1: Current prosthesis systems.

Model	**S.T.A.R. (Fig. 4.1)**	**SALTO (Fig. 4.2)**	**MOBILITY (Fig. 4.3)**	**HINTEGRA (Fig. 4.4)**	**ESKA (Fig. 4.5)**	**TARIC (Fig. 4.6)**
Author	Dr. H. Kofoed	Dr. M. Bonnin, Dr. J.A. Colombier, Dr. T. Judet	Dr. P. Rippstein, Dr. P. Wood, Dr. C. Coetzee	Prof. B. Hintermann, Dr. G. Derymaeker, Dr. R. Viladot, Dr. P. Diebold	Prof. J. Rudigier	Prof. S. Rehart, Prof. B. Fink, Dr. S. Schill, Dr. K. Schenck
Distribution	WALDEMAR LINK GmbH & Co. KG	Tornier GmbH (Burscheid)	DePuy Orthopedics	Plus Orthopedics	ESKA-Implants	Implantcast GmbH
Year of development	1990	1997	2005	2000	1990	2005
Prosthesis design	Three-compartment model	Three-compartment model	Three-compartment model, spherical talus/inlay component	Three-compartment model	Three-compartment model	Three-compartment model
Metal	Chrome-cobalt	Chrome-cobalt	Cobalt-chrome	Chrome-cobalt	Cobalt-chrome-*molybdenum*	Chrome-cobalt-*molybdenum*
Sliding core	UHMW polyethylene	UHMW polyethylene	UHMW polyethylene	UHMW polyethylene	UHMW polyethylene	UHMW polyethylene
Surface coating	HX® (calcium phosphate) on pure titanium, since 1999 double coating	Hydroxyapatite on titanium	Porocoat	Hydroxyapatite on porous titanium	Spongiosa metal® II	cpTi pure titanium
Approach to ankle	Ventral	Ventral	Ventral	Ventral	Lateral, medial	Ventral

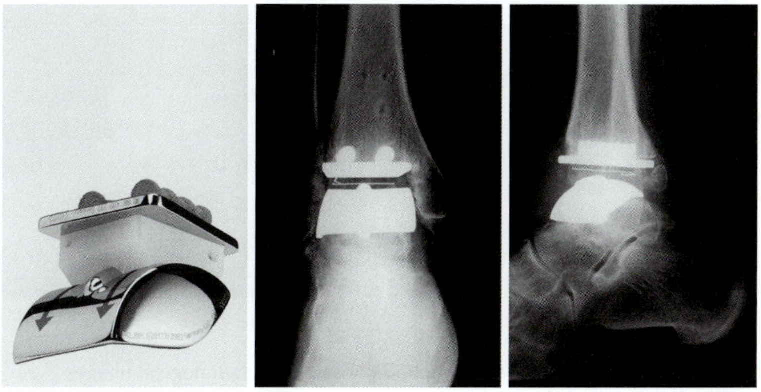

(a) (b) (c)

Fig. 4.1: S.T.A.R. prosthesis; (a) model view, (b, c) radiological images.

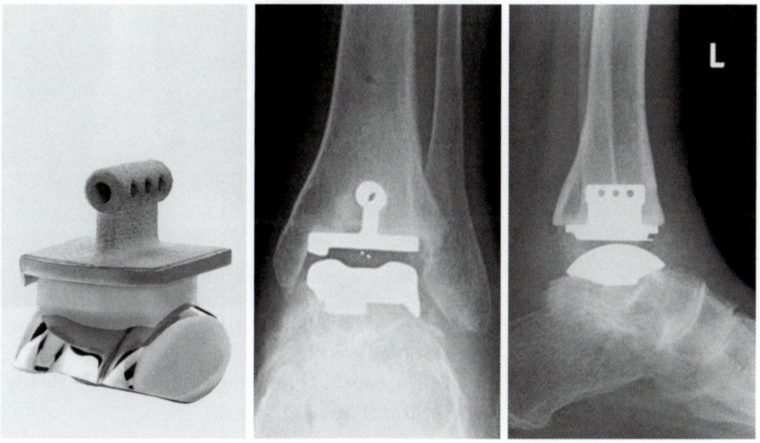

(a) (b) (c)

Fig. 4.2: SALTO prosthesis; (a) model view, (b, c) radiological images.

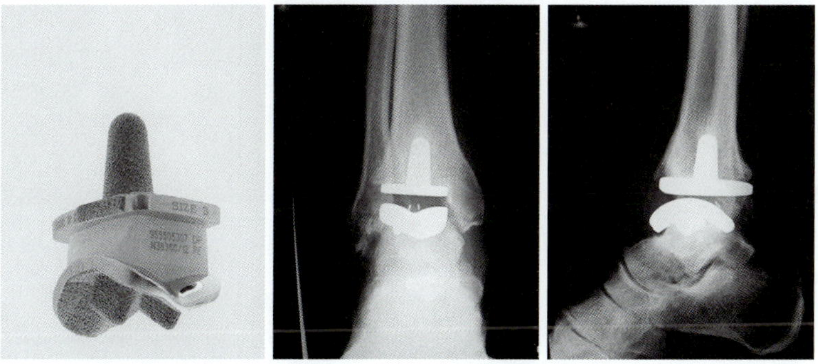

(a) (b) (c)

Fig. 4.3: MOBILITY prosthesis; (a) model view, (b, c) radiological images.

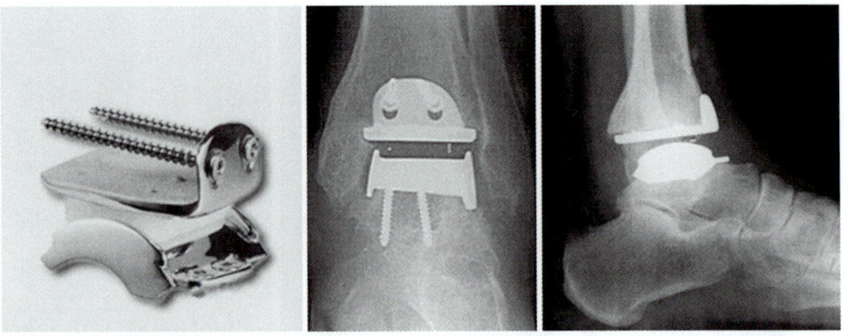

(a) (b) (c)

Fig. 4.4: HINTEGRA prosthesis; (a) model view, (b, c) radiological images (with the kind permission of Prof. B. Hintermann, Canton Hospital Liestal).

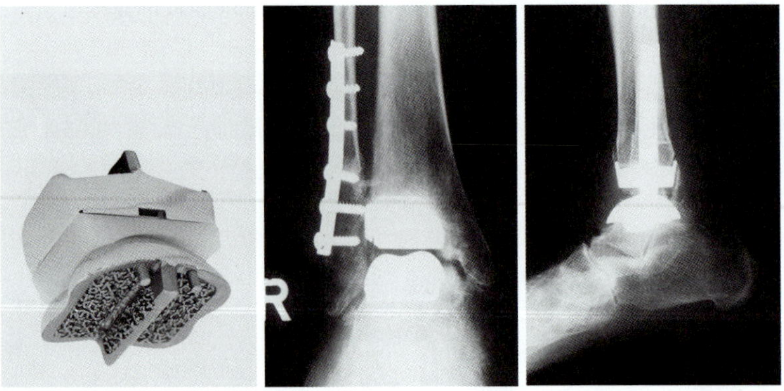

(a) (b) (c)

Fig. 4.5: ESKA prosthesis; (a) model view, (b, c) radiological images, (c) clearly visible fibular osteosynthesis after transfibular approach.

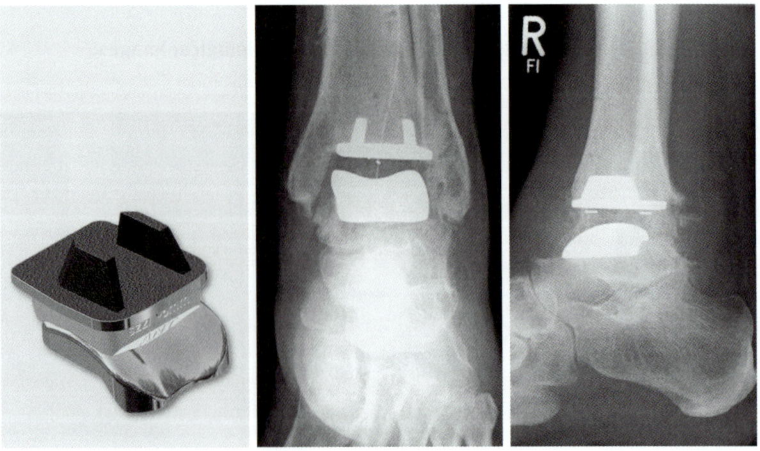

(a) (b) (c)

Fig. 4.6: TARIC prosthesis; (a) model view, (b, c) radiological images.

4.4 Indication/Contraindication

Not every clinical picture and not every patient is suitable for endoprosthetic treatment. Something that a few years ago still represented the worst diagnosis can today be treated with improved implants and optimized surgical techniques.

Not every clinical picture or every patient suitable for endoprosthesis

By far the most common indication for endoprosthetic treatment is secondary, post-traumatic arthrosis (Fig. 4.7).

Main indication: secondary, post-traumatic arthrosis

In the last few years a steady increase in patients has been observed, which can be attributed to a rise in sporting activities, even in older patients. Post-traumatically changed ankles are often accompanied by instability of the ligaments and axial malalignment, which absolutely must be considered during later surgical treatment. Furthermore, in many cases, limited movement in the upper ankle is found with secondary contraction of the flexors. Additionally, these patients often need a percutaneous Achilles tenotomy to attain the ability to perform a functional dorsal extension and extensive arthrolysis. Moreover necessary metal removal is necessary after previous operations (Fig. 4.7)

Steady increase in patients owing to rise in sporting activity

Often instability of the ligament and axial malalignment

Limited movement with secondary flexor contractions

Percutaneous Achilles tenotomy, arthrolysis, metal removal necessary if appropriate

In the early days of ankle endoprosthetics, rheumatics comprised the largest group of patients (Fig. 4.8). At the time of implantation they show well-preserved movement and in most cases normal axis and stable ligament conditions. Because of long-term pain anamnesis, these patients have a good outcome in relation to pain reduction and subjective satisfaction. Sometimes the changed bone condition can lead to problems in implant fixation. Furthermore, a possible long-term medication must be considered and if necessary discontinued at the time of the operation (immunosuppressives).

Rheumatics the largest group of patients

Good outcome in pain reduction and subjective satisfaction

Occasional problems in implant fixation

Consideration of long-term medication

As in patients with rheumatoid arthritis the adjacent joints (subtalar, talonavicular) are often also affected, this be given special attention. For these patients arthrodesis is the unfavorable alternative, as it can subsequently result in rapid progression of the degeneration in the adjacent joints owing to overloading.

Adjacent joints often affected

Arthrodesis unfavorable alternative

Primary arthrosis (Fig. 4.9), on the other hand, is rare and not regarded as a discrete entity by some authors. Not enough is known about the causes of this disease. A stronger load over a longer period is discussed. With them, malalignments (varus, valgus) are often found, with the consequent asymmetrical wear of the joint cartilage. A premature treatment of the malalignment, e.g., by corrective osteotomies, can occasionally delay or even prevent endoprosthetic treatment. In the last few years, with this aspect too, a steady increase in patients also been observed.

Primary arthrosis rare

Common malalignments with asymmetrical wearing of the joint cartilage

Delay/prevention of the prosthesis implantation owing to premature treatment of malalignments

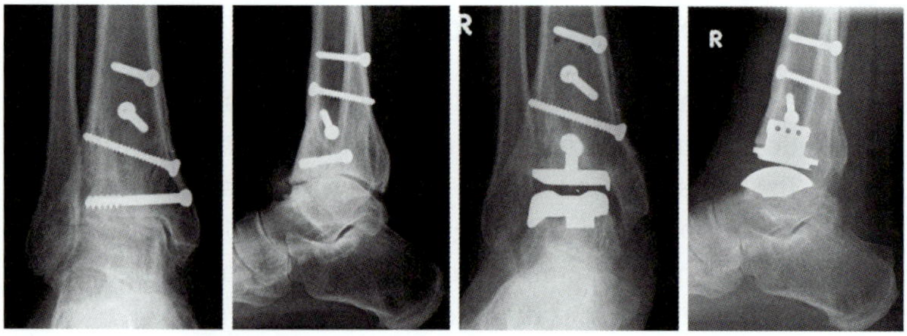

(a) (b) (c) (d)

Fig. 4.7: Post-traumatic ankle arthrosis; (a, b) preoperative image with clear articular surface destruction especially laterally, at the subchondrally placed screw, (c, d) radiological follow-up six weeks postoperatively after implantation of a SALTO endoprosthesis.

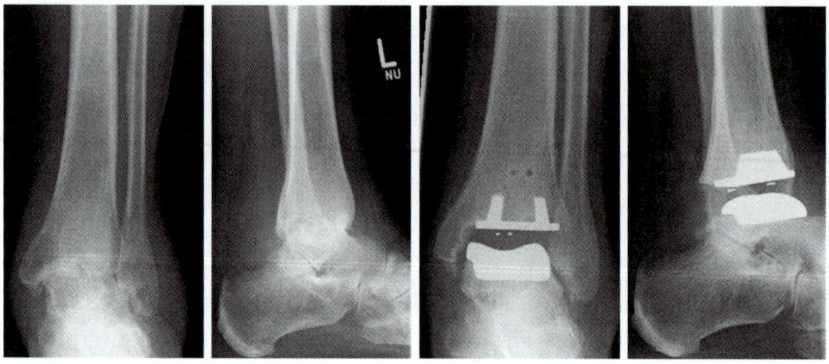

(a) (b) (c) (d)

Fig. 4.8: Secondary ankle prosthesis in rheumatoid arthritis; (a, b) preoperative findings, (c, d) radiological follow-up six weeks postoperatively after implantation of a TARIC endoprosthesis.

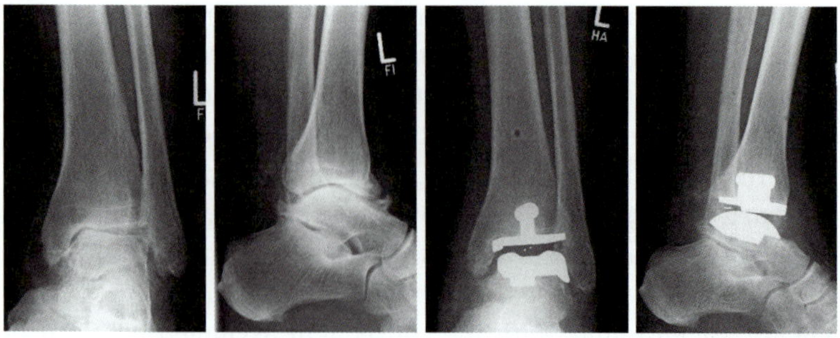

(a) (b) (c) (d)

Fig. 4.9: Primary arthrosis with varus malalignment, no trauma is noted in the anamnesis; (a, b) preoperative radiological images, (c, d) radiological follow-up six weeks postoperatively after implantation of a SALTO endoprosthesis.

4.4.1 Patient Selection

Not every patient is equally suitable for an endoprosthetic treatment. In addition to the careful clinical evaluation and medical history a basic social and professional history is necessary.

Not every patient suitable for endoprosthetic treatment

Medical history, basic social and professional history necessary

Patients who do not understand and/or do not want to comply with the therapy and after-care program should only in exceptional cases be provided with an endoprosthesis. Sporting interests and professional requirements must be taken into account and be included in the treatment planning. In this way patients with a great professional burden (construction workers, etc.) should be informed about alternative treatment methods such as arthrodesis.

Types of contact sports with recurrent compression and distortion loads ("stop and go") also represent a contraindication to endoprosthetic treatment.

Contraindication: types of contact sports

Whether the patient's weight has an influence on the long-term outcome has to date not been clearly resolved. In our clinic this circumstance does not currently represent a contraindication. In these cases, we try to use larger implants and higher inlays.

Influence of weight on long-term outcome unresolved

Today, the patient's age plays a rather inferior role in patient selection. While previously an endoprosthesis was only implanted in older patients, the spectrum of indications has today also been extended to young, sporty and active patients with arthrosis.

Patient age insignificant

4.4.2 Bone Situation

Good bone condition is an important basic requirement in the field of endoprosthetics. A secure primary fixation is essential for adequate secondary osseointegration. Pronounced bone defects, therefore, represent a contraindication (Fig. 4.10). In this cases primary arthrodesis is the treatment of choice.

Contraindication: pronounced bone defects

Primary arthrodesis treatment of choice

Both isolated (talar, tibial) and combined defect zones are to be found.

Isolated or combined defect zones

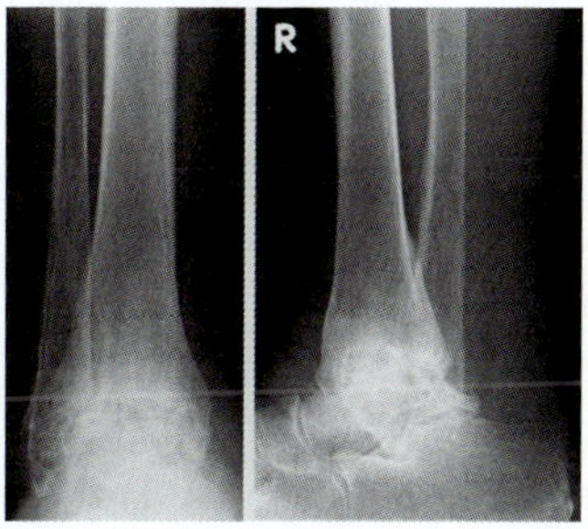

(a) (b)

Fig. 4.10: Combined arthrosis of the upper and lower ankle with pronounced bone destruction and defect zones. The zones of necrosis in the talus reach up to the neck area.

Talar necrosis up to 50 % tolerable if necessary

Only a low level of cortical defects tolerable

Talar necrosis of up to 50 % is tolerable in exceptional cases and under certain requirements (Fig. 4.24). Here, defects are filled and bridged with a spongiosa graft.

As 90 % of the application of force on the tibial components of the endoprosthesis runs over the cortex, a lower level of defects is tolerated here. For this reason intraoperative tibial resection should also be carried out very sparingly.

Contraindication: severe osteoporosis

Severe osteoporosis represents a contraindication to ankle endoprosthetics.

4.4.3 Ligamentous Situation

Implantation impeded by instability at the ankle

Ligament injuries often underestimated and inadequately treated

Contraindication: ligament insufficiencies that cannot be reconstructed

Lateral ligaments: various reconstruction techniques

Medial ligament complex: reconstruction complex, lower chances of success

Instability at the ankle favors not only the formation of arthrosis at the ankle, but also impedes later endoprosthesis implantation. Ligament injuries are often underestimated, trivialized, and inadequately treated. The tibiotalar congruence compensates for the eversion and inversion forces, while the ligament complex stabilizes the rotational and a.p. translational forces. Modern three-component endoprostheses do not exhibit any constraining. Insufficiencies after endoprosthesis implantation can therefore lead to instability of the joint, which can result in non-directional application of force and inappropriate loading. This again causes unilateral overloading, which can lead to premature inlay wear or to malalignment and fractures. If ligamentous insufficiencies cannot be reconstructed, this is regarded as a contraindication. For the lateral ligaments various reconstruction techniques are available. Conversely, the reconstruction of the medial ligament complex is more complex and has, especially in cases of chronic instability (valgus deformity), lower chances of success.

4.4.4 General Contraindications

General contraindications:
- Florid or recent infections

Prevention of hematogenous seeding

Florid or recent infections are clearly regarded as contraindications. If a preoperative rise in the inflammatory markers (CRP, leukocytes) is shown, screening (dental chart, ENT, etc.) should be carried out. Hematogenous seeding must be prevented. The postinfectious state after less recent joint infections do not in our view represent any contraindication if at the time of the operation no suspected clinical or paraclinical infection exists. A postoperative antibiotic screen over the duration of the in-patient stay can be implemented.

In the case of extensive soft-tissue defects combined with muscular and ligamentous insufficiencies a thorough, narrow definition of indications must be made. This is to be considered particularly in patients after several interventions in the lower leg and foot (e.g., after severe trauma), as here the degree of perfusion is often defective or ambiguous. When in doubt, radiological angiography (DSA, angio-MRT) is recommended.

Narrow definition of indications in the case of combined soft-tissue defects and muscular/ligamentous insufficiencies
When in doubt radiological angiography

As mentioned before, adequate bone condition is a basic requirement for successful prosthesis implantation. Thus, pronounced bone defects are classified as an absolute contraindication. These include among others body of talar necrosis/defects >50 % and bone sequelae of peripheral neuropathies (Charcot foot).

- Pronounced bone defects

Situations after arthrodesis with a longer lasting lack of movement of the upper ankle and a resulting insufficiency of the tendons and musculature are usually classed as contraindications and should only be carried out as an absolute exception (Fig. 4.11),

- Situation after arthrodesis with longer lasting lack of movement of the upper ankle and insufficiency of the tendons/musculature

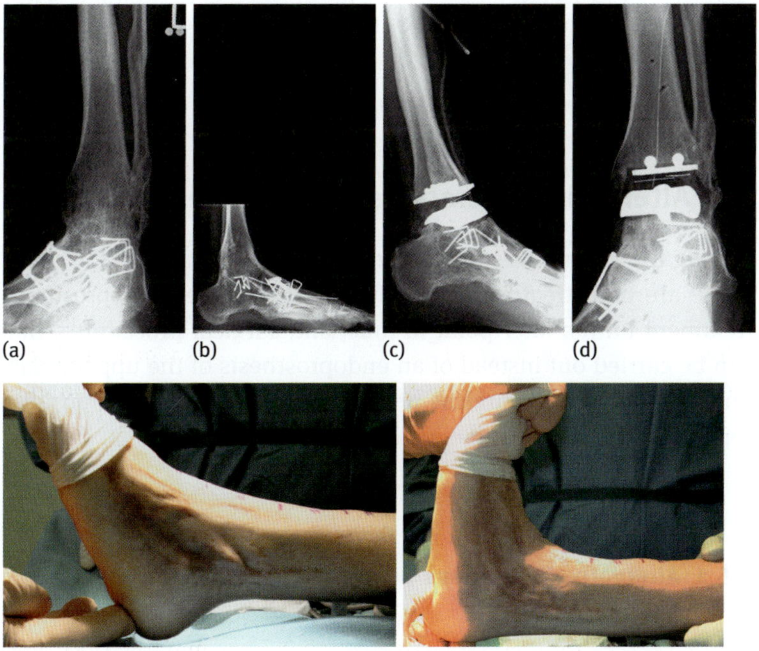
(a) (b) (c) (d) (e) (f)

Fig. 4.11: De-arthrodesis after arthrodesis of the upper and lower ankles as well as a partial mid-foot arthrodesis. A physiological flexing movement of the foot was no longer possible and the patient could no longer manage in this situation. The de-arthrodesis was the last resort before amputation. (a, b) Preoperative radiological images, (c, d) postoperative radiological images after implantation of a S.T.A.R. endoprosthesis, (e, f) intraoperative clinical findings (extension/flexion).

after intensived conversations with the patient, and in specialized centers. Statements about the outcome, especially in relation to postoperative mobility, cannot or can only inadequately be encountered.

General contraindications

General contraindications to an ankle endoprosthesis are:
- General cardiovascular contraindications to an operation
- Clinically significant arterial perfusion defects
- High-grade, movement-limiting arthrosis of the upper ankle
- Non-reconstructive ligamentous insufficiencies
- Extensive bone and soft-tissue defects after previous operations
- Patients who cannot understand or adhere to the after-care program (compliance)
- Florid or recent infections in the operative area
- Systemic infections
- Charcot foot and relevant neurological diseases
- Uncorrectable malalignment
- Talar necrosis with defects of the talar dome more than 50 %
- Heavy physical performance requirements (professional and in sport)

4.5 Alternative Operations at the Upper Ankle

Alternatives to endoprosthetic replacement of the upper ankle

Among the alternatives to endoprosthetic replacement of the upper ankle are both treatment procedures, which defer endoprosthetic treatment until a later point in time, and surgical procedures, that can be carried out instead of an endoprosthesis of the upper ankle. Furthermore, other surgical procedures come into question after removal of an upper ankle endoprosthesis.

4.5.1 Alternative Operations Before Ankle Endoprosthesis Implantation

Causes of circumscribed defects with consequent arthrosis of the upper ankle

Here, operations shall be discussed that can be used in the case of already clearly recognizable cartilage defects, without the joint stiffening or being replaced by an artificial joint. Causes of the circumscribed defects with consequent arthrosis of the upper ankle are post-traumatic cartilage defects, osteochondrosis dissecans, aseptic osteonecrosis of the talus, and varus arthrosis. Patients between 20 and 50 years of age are predominantly affected. Some defects are already clearly recognizable on the X-ray as circumscribed osteochondrosis dissecans or unilaterally as the start of arthrosis. They have a worse prognosis than defects that can only be seen on MRT. Here, the treatment with the use of arthroscopy, synovectomy, OATS plastic (osteochondral autologous transplantation) or chondrocyte transplantation can be carried out.

On the X-ray recognizable defects with worse prognosis than those recognizable on MRT

Treatment possibilities

In the last few years the performance of supramalleolar osteotomies has proven to be of value as another therapeutic possibility. The indications are similar to those for tibial head osteotomy in the preparation to place an endoprosthesis implantation. Supramalleolar osteotomies are particularly applied in idiopathic varus arthrosis of the upper ankle, and occasionally in valgus arthrosis too. In addition, these interventions are debated in patients who carry out hard physical work, marked talar necrosis, as well as obesity or morbid obesity, in which an artificial joint replacement is very reluctantly pursued.

Another therapeutic possibility: supramalleolar osteotomies

Further indications

Osteotomies are often carried out in the case of varus or valgus changes in the hindfoot of more than 15°. These axial deviations can appear on the one hand within the upper ankle between the talus and tibia, but on the other in the distal lower leg owing to a post-traumatic change in the tibia.

Osteotomies often in the case of varus and valgus changes in the hindfoot

In these patients correction can be achieved by removal of a wedge of bone with a lateral base (varus arthrosis) or medial base (valgus arthrosis). For osteosynthesis after these osteotomies special locking plates are available. As in closed wedge osteotomy (for varus arthrosis) a piece of the fibula must be removed at the same time, fibular osteosynthesis can also be used for fixation of the osteotomy (Fig. 4.12).

Performance of osteotomies

In osteotomies the preservation of a biomechanical load axis must also be heeded. As well as the technique with removal of a bone wedge (closed wedge) the possibility of an added axial correc-

Important: Preservation of a biomechanical load axis

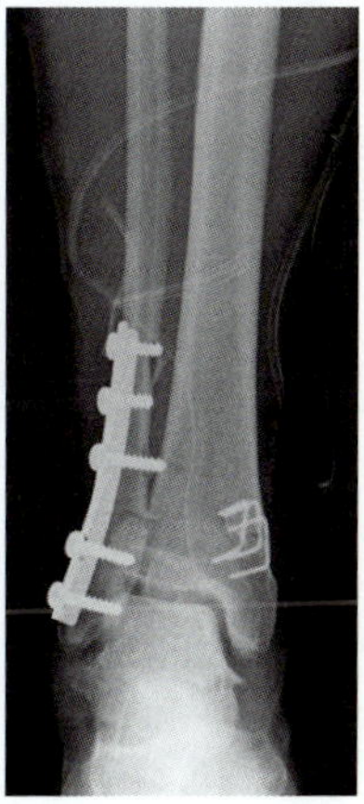

Fig. 4.12: Radiological image after lateral closed wedge osteotomy in varus arthrosis of the upper ankle. Fibular and medial staple osteosynthesis for stabilization of the osteotomy.

tion (open wedge). Here, the fixation is carried out over the special osteosynthesis plates.

Secondary osteotomy for axis straightening much more complicated

It is known that preoperative axial deviation s at the ankle significantly worsen the treatment results after endoprosthesis (secondary prosthesis dislocations, malleolus fractures, loss of correction). This is indicative of the performance of osteotomies as a preparatory intervention before endoprosthesis implantation. In our experience, it is less complicated – but possible – to carry out a secondary osteotomy axial straightening after endoprosthetic treatment.

Correction osteotomies with simultaneously performed joint-enhancing measures

Corrective osteotomies can be expanded by simultaneously performed joint-enhancing measures. Thus, we carry out in one stage drilling of the sclerotized joint parts at the talus or its microfractures. The ablation of ventral osteophytes and the performance of a synovectomy are almost obligatory if significant inflammation is present.

4.5.2 Alternatives to Total Endoprosthesis

Stiffening of the upper ankles only real alternative to total endoprosthesis

Today, stiffening no longer the gold standard

While 20 years ago good results after interpositional arthroplasty and denervation were still being reported, it has gone very quiet around these interventions. Today, stiffening of the upper ankle is seen as the only real alternative. In our opinion it can no longer be denoted the gold standard. While in the Orthopedic University Clinic of Magdeburg around 100–150 ankle endoprosthesis are inserted per year, we only carry out 10–15 primary arthrodeses of the ankle. The biggest disadvantage of arthrodesis is that the complaints increase rather than decrease over a period of years when mobilization of the adjacent joints comes about and/or secondary (stiffening) arthrosis occurs. Hence, younger patients with arthrodesis have a rather bad long-term prognosis and therefore benefit from a total endoprosthesis.

Younger patients with arthrodesis have a rather bad long-term prognosis

Primary fixation significant for the success of isolated arthrodesis

Significant for the success of isolated arthrodesis of the upper ankle is the primary fixation. Here, the fixation is conducted with screws for good results. Furthermore, arthrodesis with the use of external fixation, retrograde interlocking nails, and arthroscopically supported techniques is possible.

Various techniques for cartilage resection of the upper ankle

There are also various techniques for cartilage resection of the upper ankle. The cartilage resection can take place during open surgery with the use of oscillating saws through resection of the parts close to the joint, but also through the arthroscopic removal of the joint cartilage. Comparative, prospective, randomized studies on these individual methods are not available; thus, their use depends on the personal experience of the surgeon.

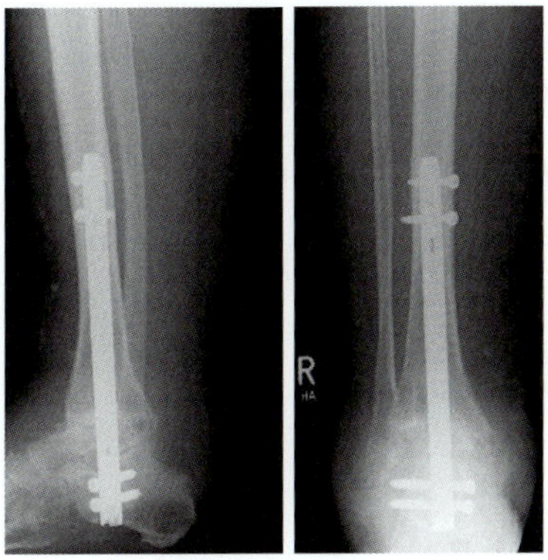

Fig. 4.13: Postoperative radiological image after combined lower and upper ankle arthrodesis by means of retrograde interlocking nails.

In some cases the endoprosthesis must be removed secondarily. Occasionally continuation is intolerably painful. More often secondary loosening and osteonecrosis occur, especially in the talar area. One of the most frequent causes of explantation is surely infection. What they all have in common is that they usually lead to a substance defect in the joint area. If the lower ankle is at the same time so damaged that it should also be stiffened, the treatment is technically the easiest. In these cases retrograde interlocking nails are used (Fig. 4.13) that can be distally fixed both in the calcaneal area and in the talar area. Furthermore, the possibility exists of proximal dynamization after six weeks in order to achieve sufficient compression. If substance defects are present, an autologous spongiosa graft should be carried out under aseptic conditions. For questionable infections it is recommended to perform this in a second intervention.

Secondary removal of the endoprosthesis

Causes:
- Rarely: intolerable pain
- Secondary loosening
- Osteonecrosis
- Infection

It is of course completely mistaken to believe that just as good a functional result can be achieved with secondary arthrodesis after removal of an ankle endoprosthesis as with a primary stiffening of the upper ankle.

Secondary arthrodesis with worse functional result than primary stiffening

4.6 Surgical Technique

A large part of the implants used today are implanted via a standardized ventral approach. An exception to this is provided by the AGILITY prosthesis, which requires an additional incision over the distal fibula for stabilization of the syndesmosis. The ESKA prosthesis is implanted entirely via a lateral, transfibular approach (Fig. 4.5).

Implantation usually via a standardized ventral approach

15–30 minutes before the operation an antibiotic screen should be put in place. The optional application of a tourniquet may follow. By doing this a good overview during the operation can be

Antibiotic screen before surgery

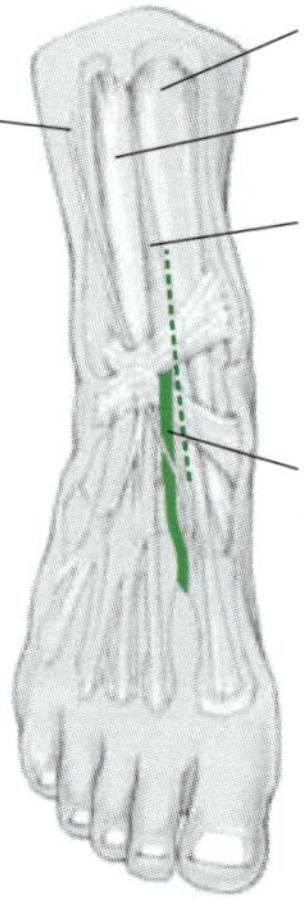

Fig. 4.14: Anatomical landmarks for the ventral approach to the ankle.

Optional: application of a tourniquet

achieved. However, for the purposes of prolonged interventions timing problems can come about, which make it necessary to open up the tourniquet during the operation.

Incision technique

The skin incision should not be too small (0.1 m–0.15 m) and in normal cases quickly lead over the talonavicular joint. After subcutaneous preparation and representation of the retinaculum, the incision is made lengthways on the periphery of the tendon of the M. tibialis anterior (Fig. 4.14).

Surgical procedure

After representation of the joint the articular capsule is resected and any possible ventral osteophytes present are removed. Depending on the prosthesis model used the tibial precision instruments are positioned and anchored. Additionally, tibial resection

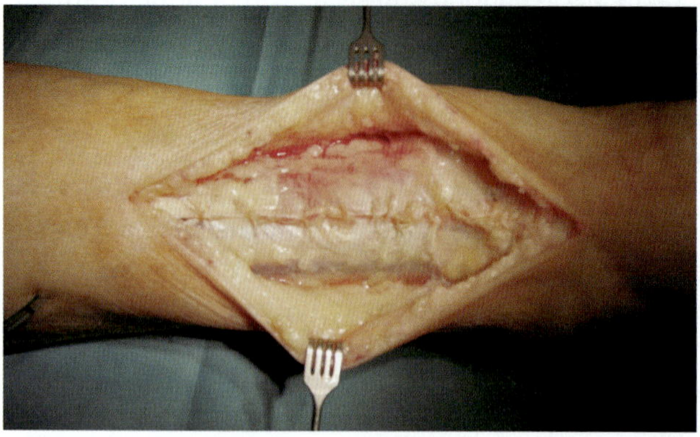

Fig. 4.15: Intraoperative site after subtle sealing of the retinaculum with the suture button technique. Thus, the danger of the formation of a subcutaneous hematoma is reduced.

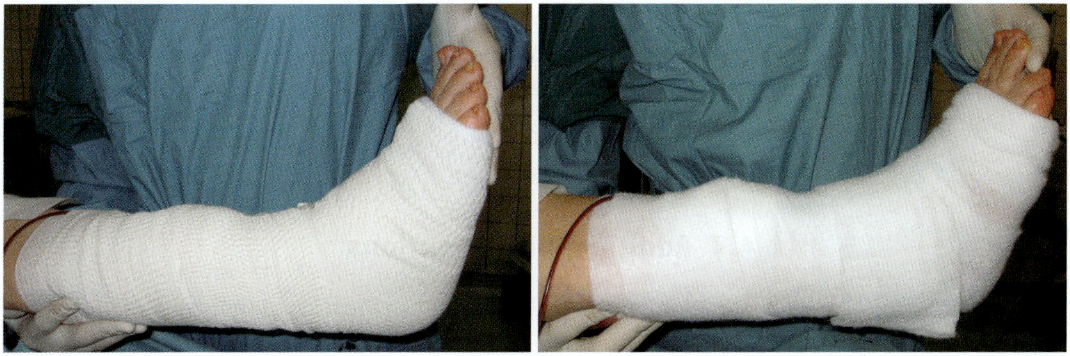

(a) (b)

Fig. 4.16: (a) Postoperative wound dressing with cotton under-padding (b).

takes place. After removal of the resected tissue the talar resection plane is referred to and consequently prepared with the use of saw guides for the talar components. With the use of test components the correct place and interaction can now be checked. Consequently, the original implants are inserted without cement – with the use of the press-fit technique. After repeated function checks and intensive lavage a drain was inserted and the wound closed in layers.

Subtle sealing of the retinaculum

In our clinic special value is placed on the subtle sealing of the retinaculum. It is always carried out using a suture button and is continued for as long until the retinaculum is sealed "watertight" (Fig. 4.15). Thus, hemorrhage into the subcutaneous soft tissue and the consequent danger of wound healing disorders are minimized. To check, the tourniquet is opened and any possible dehiscences are sutured.

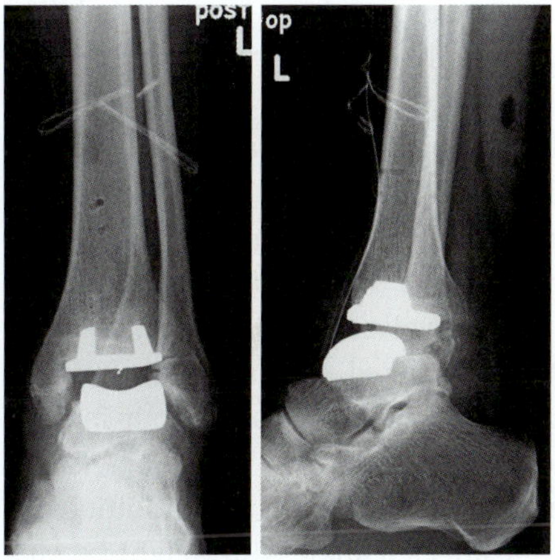

Fig. 4.17: Postoperative radiological image after implantation of ankle endoprosthesis (TARIC).

End of the operation

After subcutaneous and skin suturing a wound bandage with cotton under-padding is applied (Fig. 4.16). A postoperative X-ray check in two planes is standard (Fig. 4.17).

4.7 Additional Interventions

Higher complication and/ or revision rate through greater malalignment in the frontal plane

Correct diagnosis and treatment of the malalignment necessary

For a long time, malalignment in the area of the ankle of more than 10° in the frontal plane was a contraindication to implantation of an ankle prosthesis. Some publications prove that greater malalignment in the frontal plane, and varus malalignment in particular, is afflicted with a high complication and/or revision rate after total endoprosthesis of the upper ankle (UA-TEP). To expand the spectrum of indications for the endoprosthesis it is therefore necessary to diagnose this malalignment correctly and treat accordingly in order to ultimately guarantee an axially correct prosthesis implantation.

Many different surgical techniques for stabilizing the ankle using endoprosthesis

Raised surgical risk with necessary additional operations

Some additional interventions have a longer rehabilitation phase

The spectrum of the various surgical techniques for stabilizing the ankle in connection with an endoprosthesis ranges from soft tissue stabilizing in the capsule area and ligament structures, e.g., by medial release, to ligament grafts and/or tendon transfer, up to osteotomies and correction arthrodesis of the adjacent joints. Thus, it now seems possible to successfully treat ankles with great malalignment long-term using an endoprosthesis; however, the limits are certainly fluid and depend considerably on the surgeon's wealth of experience. Through necessary additional operations the direct surgical risk with regard to complications is indeed raised and/or some additional interventions require a longer rehabilitation phase. Therefore, this should all be thoroughly discussed with the patient in advance.

Type and extent of the correction dependent on localization and deformity

Difference between flexible and fixed malalignment

The type and extent of the correction to be carried out depend quite considerably on the localization and the deformity. In the frontal plane the malalignment can appear isolated on the one hand to the tibiotalar joint but on the other to the subtalar joint. Not uncommonly, both joints are involved. Furthermore, we must differentiate between flexible and/or fixed malalignment. Preoperatively, a basic clinical examination must be carried out in each case. The evaluation of the joint stasis in the standing patient involving standing on tiptoe is very important in this. Additionally, in a.p. projection an X-ray of the affected ankle with weight-bearing on the foot is necessary anyway. In some cases long leg radiographs are needed for evaluation of the joint axes.

4.7.1 Tibiotalar Malalignment (Varus/Valgus)

Valgus malalignment in the upper ankle is rather rare compared with varus malalignment and can often be reoriented by axially correct implantation of an endoprosthesis alone. Varus arthrosis occurs far more frequently (Fig. 4.18).

Valgus malalignment rare, varus arthrosis much more common

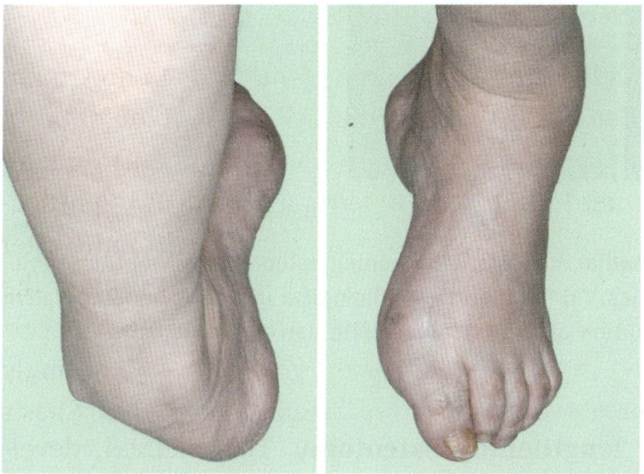

Fig. 4.18: Clinical image of varus malalignment of the upper ankle.

With regard to etiology, we must distinguish between idiopathic varus arthrosis of the upper ankle (often bilateral, preferably in men) and the post-traumatic status with chronic outer ligament insufficiency. While the former is often firmly fixed in the varus position, can no longer be corrected and thus leads to an unphysiological gait on the outer edge of the foot, with the post-traumatic lateral unstable ankle a good chance of passive correction is shown. Radiologically, in both cases there is a medially stressed tibiotalar loss of substance in both joint partners with varus tilting of the talus in the ankle mortise. The tibiotalar angle, i.e., the talar tilt in relation to the long axis of the tibia on a.p. projection under weight-bearing is regarded as an approximate measure of deformity, whereas the subtalar components are not taken into account.

Difference between idiopathic varus arthrosis and post-traumatic status with chronic outer ligament insufficiency

The correction possibilities are presented below.

Medial release. With the so-called medial release the contracting ligamentous structures (deltoid ligament) should be loosened. For this reason the insertion areas of the deltoid ligament are detached mostly with the use of saws or chisels subperiosteally under simultaneous valgus stress on the hindfoot. Nevertheless, experience has shown that only smaller malalignments of up to 10° can be compensated for with this method. Possible complications such as vascular and axonal injuries (tarsal tunnel) can occur with this method.

Compensation for smaller malalignment of up to around 10° by medial release

Complications: vascular and axonal injuries

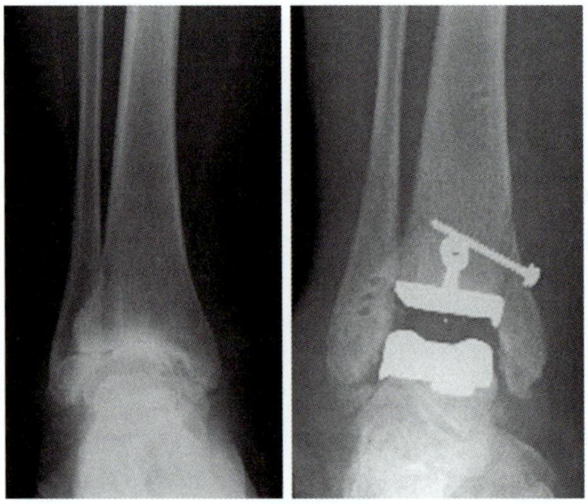

(a) (b)

Fig. 4.19: One-stage medial malleolar lengthening osteotomy within the scope of ankle endoprosthetics. (a) Preoperative radiological image, (b) postoperative radiological image: fixation of the osteotomy with use of osteosynthesis screws.

Medial malleolar lengthening osteotomy: good, secure possibility of correction with existing fixed varus deformities

Medial malleolar lengthening osteotomy. This method, developed by von Doets, offers a good, secure possibility of correction in existing fixed varus deformities. In this method an extensive osteotomy is carried out in the area of the medial malleolus directly next to the boundary of the medial tibial plate. It can now be distalized and refixed to the malleolus with its usually contracting ligamentous insertions (Fig. 4.19). The extent of the distalization is usually determined by horizontal (test) prosthesis and can thus be relatively precisely ascertained.

Complications: pseudarthrosis, fractures

Possible complications are seen in the occurrence of pseudarthrosis and/or fractures. The patient is also informed of a prolonged rehabilitation period.

Reconstruction of the outer ligaments treatment option in the case of flexible varus malalignment and lateral ligament insufficiency

Outer ligament grafts. In flexible varus malalignments with a passive possibility of correction and proven lateral ligament insufficiency, the reconstruction of the outer ligaments represents a possible treatment option. On the one hand, this can be performed via tendon grafts (e.g., peroneus longus transfer) or by inserting so-called artificial ligaments. Indeed, these procedures are often suitable only in combination with other techniques, as at least partially contracted conditions are usually present. On the other hand, tendon grafts or tendon replacement operations require a longer phase of immobilization postoperatively, which can have a detrimental effect directly connected to an endoprosthesis implantation. Last but not least, it also indicates the necessity for a second skin incision, with the potential danger of the occurrence of wound healing disorders.

Longer phase of immobilization

Tibialis anterior transposition. The transfer of the tibialis anterior tendon to the lateral edge of the foot represents a relatively new procedure related to upper ankle endoprosthetics. As an established procedure in children and neuro-orthopedic corrective interventions, it was picked up by Hamel and modified in the context of ankle endoprosthetics and/or their revision. Combined with other procedures these methods seem to represent, at least in the short to middle term, a vital factor in the rebalancing of the joint axis.

Tibialis anterior transposition vital factor for the rebalancing of the joint axis

4.7.2 Subtalar Malalignment (Varus/Valgus)

While isolated varus malalignment in the subtalar joint are rather rare, valgus malalignments are often the end result of an acquired hard pes plano valgus with loss of the medial foot arch supports. In order to achieve a good result for the endoprosthesis, subtalar malalignment must be heeded and corrected before or at the time of the implantation of an ankle endoprosthesis.

Valgus malalignment often the result of an acquired hard pes plano valgus
Correction of a subtalar malalignment before or at the time of implantation

Medializing calcaneal osteotomy. The valgus malalignment of the hindfoot can in most cases be corrected well by a medializing calcaneal shift osteotomy. Here, via a second small lateral approach directly behind the course of the peroneal tendon the osteotomy is performed intraoperatively, so that the tuber calcanei can then be temporarily shifted one or two centimeters medially. The fixation is performed as a rule by the insertion of one or two compression screws (Fig. 4.20). In cases of stronger medialization the lateral edge should be flattened in the area of malalignment of

Correction of a valgus malalignment of the hindfoot by medializing calcaneal shift osteotomy

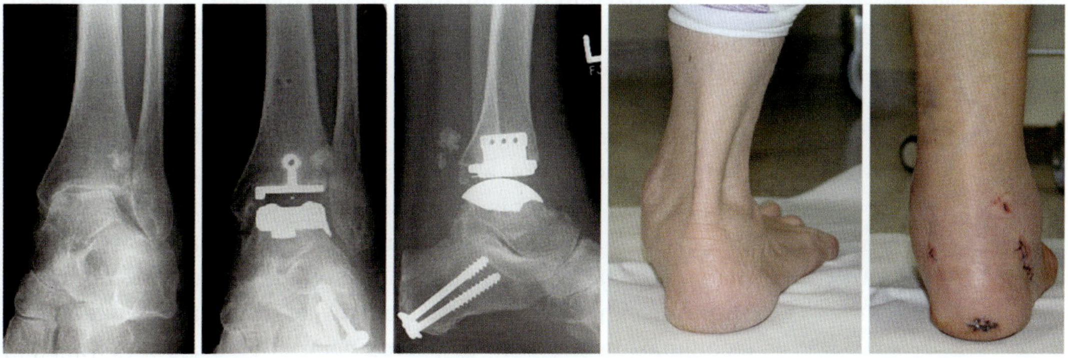

(a) (b) (c) (d) (e)

Fig. 4.20: Medializing calcaneal osteotomy in cases of valgized hindfoot position;
(a) preoperative radiological image, (b, c) postoperative radiological images, (d) preoperative clinical image, (e) postoperative clinical image.

the osteotomy in order to prevent pressure discomfort. Also, the inserted screws in the calcaneal area can occasionally be troublesome; thus, they have to be removed after healing of the osteotomy.

Correction of a varus malalignment of the heel by lateralized calcaneal shift osteotomy

Valgizing calcaneal osteotomy. In varus malalignment of the heel a lateralizing calcaneal shift osteotomy can be carried out in order to minimize the varus moment on the ankle by the lateralizing effect on the Achilles tendon. The osteotomy also takes place via a second lateral skin incision dorsal to the peroneal tendon. By removing a small wedge with a lateral base and simultaneous lateral shift of the tuber calcanei the heel can be valgized correspondingly. Here, too, protruding bone should be removed to prevent pressure discomfort. Alternatively, a z-shaped osteotomy, as described by Hintermann, can be carried out.

Alternative: z-shaped osteotomy according to Hintermann

Correction of severe flat foot deformities in rheumatoid arthritis with hindfoot arthrodesis

Hindfoot arthrodesis. The indication for carrying out hindfoot arthrodesis results almost exclusively in severe flat foot deformities in the context of rheumatoid arthritis. In the case of pronounce arthritic changes in the subtalar and talonavicular joint these can be fused to achieve stable and plantigrade foot alignment. The fusion is usually performed with the use of screw arthrodesis. If necessary, a two-stage approach is favored here, as, based on the sensitive perfusion conditions at the talus by the implanted prosthesis and the additionally incorporated osteosynthesis material, there is a potential danger of talar necrosis occurring.

Two-stage approach to prevent talar necrosis

4.7.3 Club Foot Deformity

Club deformities often in cases of post-traumatic arthrosis

In ankles fixed in the club foot position that have often been forming gradually over many years, are frequently observed in cases of post-traumatic arthrosis.

Treatment of Achilles tendon contracture at the same time as implantation of the ankle prosthesis

Achilles tendon lengthening. The total resection of the dorsal ankle capsule is not always sufficient in relation to prosthesis implantation to enable satisfactory dorsal extension of the foot. This existing Achilles tendon contracture should then be treated at the same time as the implantation of the ankle endoprosthesis. This can either be performed openly or using the percutaneous technique. In the case of percutaneous Achilles tenotomy three equal stab incisions on alternate sides are made percutaneously in the tendon area in the highly elevated leg under Achilles tendon tension, and the foot is thereby gradually redressed dorsally (Fig. 4.21).

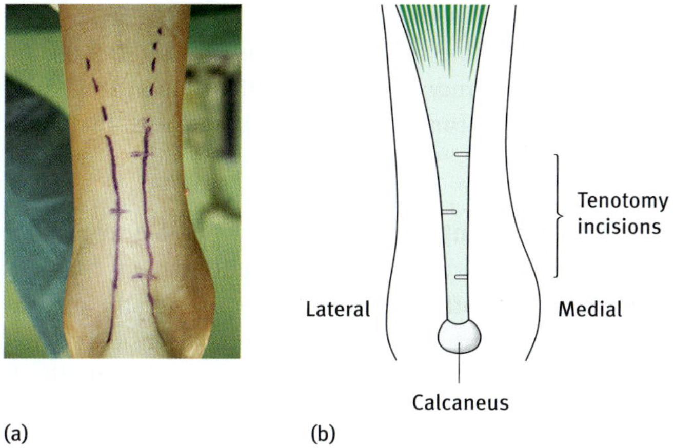

Fig. 4.21: Percutaneous, selective Achilles tenotomy; (a) intraoperative site, (b) schematic representation.

The advantage of this method certainly lies in its relatively simple technical execution. With enough experience the extent of the lengthening can be very subtly determined, since over-correction with the resulting loss of plantar flexion strength should be prevented.

Advantage: relatively simply technical execution

Venous hemorrhage and/or axonal injury (nervus suralis) must be considered as possible complications.

Complications

The sectioning of the gastrocnemius aponeurosis directly distal to the muscular insertion is named as an alternative technical procedure to percutaneous Achilles tendon lengthening. It is a matter of discussion that the plantar flexion is less affected by this method.

Alternative: sectioning of the gastrocnemius aponeurosis

Both techniques should, however, be applied in moderation in order to prevent over-correction. In general, achieving 10° dorsal extension is sufficient.

Moderate application to prevent over-correction

4.7.4 Arthrosis of the Adjacent Joints

The evaluation of the clinical relevance and thus the value of treating existing arthrosis in the adjacent joints, especially the subtalar and talonavicular joint, is difficult and is discussed controversially. For the patient's part, often only general information on painfulness in the ankle area is provided. In any case, a very specific survey of the patient with regard to pain behavior, e.g., when walking on uneven ground, should be carried out. An axially correct hindfoot position notwithstanding, the radiological presence of

Controversial discussion on the clinical relevance and treatment vale of existing arthrosis in adjacent joints

Diagnostic intra-articular injections of a local anesthetic in the subtalar and/or talonavicular joint helpful in preoperative planning

advanced arthrotic changes in the adjacent joints does not also have to involve an inevitable therapeutic consequence. Diagnostic intra-articular injections under a local anesthetic in the subtalar and/or talonavicular joint can be helpful in the preoperative planning.

Indication for arthrosis of the affected joint
- Possible complications
- Difficult/longer rehab phase

Arthrodesed joints with longer immobilization

After successful endoprosthesis implantation often unburdening of the adjacent joints, abatement of pain

In the case of persistent pain, arthrodesis of the affected adjacent joint also in the interval

Arthrodesis of the adjacent joints. In the case of the proven clinical relevance and radiologically verified arthrotic changes the indication for arthrosis of the affected joint can be given in the context of endoprosthetic treatment. However, it should be considered that the advantage of the one-stage treatment is opposed by the disadvantage of possible complications (in particular, wound healing) and/or an impeded or lengthened rehabilitation phase. While the aim of endoprosthesis implantation in the upper ankle is fast mobilization to achieve good functioning, as a rule, arthrodesed ankles require longer immobilization. Furthermore, it is indicated that after successful endoprosthesis implantation the affected adjacent joint is unburdened and thus no longer painful. If there is persistent pain the arthrodesis of the affected adjacent joint can be performed in the interval. If there are fixed deformities and existing arthrosis as well as patients with rheumatoid arthritis the (correction) arthrodesis should if necessary be performed before implantation of an ankle endoprosthesis in order to preserve a stable, plantigrade feet. In some exceptional cases it is also possible to temporarily fix the subtalar joint by anterograde insertion of two compression screws in one stage as the implantation of the endoprosthesis, whereas a debridement of the joint surfaces is then abandoned (Fig. 4.22). In the case of a partly ankylosed, painful talonavicular joint, this can be converted by inserting staples into the total ankylosis (Fig. 4.22).

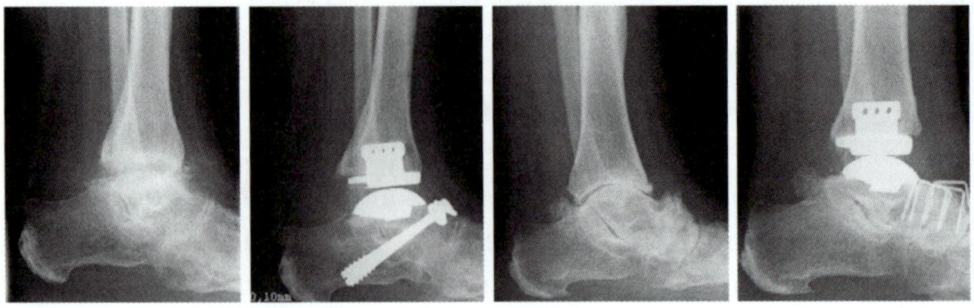

(a) (b) (c) (d)

Fig. 4.22: (a, b) Example of a one-stage endoprosthetic treatment and subtalar arthrodesis. In these cases the screws can be applied ventrally. (c, d) Example of one-stage endoprosthetic treatment and talonavicular arthrodesis using staples.

4.8 Radiological Diagnosis

Careful preoperative planning is a basic requirement for a successful intervention. To this, as well as the basic anamnesis and clinical examination a standardized radiological diagnosis is included.

Standardized radiological diagnosis

Careful preoperative planning basic requirement for successful intervention

For each patient an a.p. radiograph in the standing position and under weight-bearing are produced with 20° inner rotation and lateral projection (Fig. 4.23).

In the case of malalignment in the area of the hip or knee joint additional radiographs must be taken. Here, the long leg radiograph is an effective means of recognizing combined malalignments (Fig. 4.24). If there are further questions, e.g., rotational malalignment, CT examinations can be carried out.

Additional radiographs in the case of malalignments in the hip or knee areas

If necessary, additional CT examinations

The determination of axial malalignment is of special significance with regard to ankle endoprosthetics, since deviations from a normal axial application of force can lead to secondary revisions with above-average frequency (loosening, periprosthetic fractures). Therefore, they are bound to attract special interest during preoperative planning.

Determination of axial malalignment important for the prevention of loosening, periprosthetic fractures

MRT examinations can be carried out for special problems. The extent and localization of osteonecrosis can be thus be well evaluated (Fig. 4.25). They can give information about the bone stock. In talar necrosis, in general >50 % are dissuaded from having an endoprosthesis implantation. Furthermore, MRT enables statements to be made on the chondral composition in the context of unicompartmental joint arthrosis in cases of malalignment or post-traumatic defects. Postoperatively standard radiographs are pro

MRT diagnosis for special problems

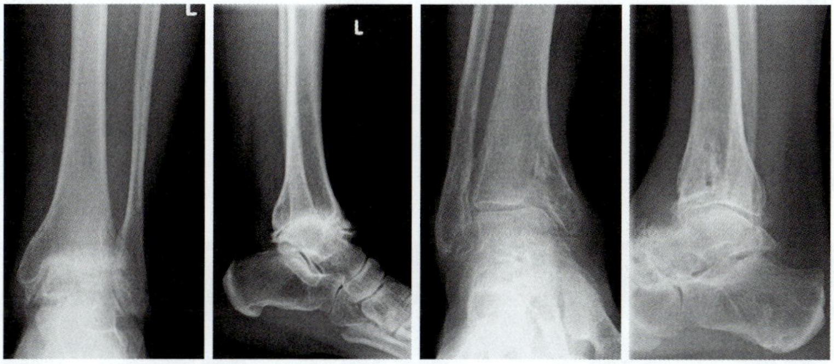

(a) (b) (c) (d)

Fig. 4.23: Standard radiographs for the preoperative preparation in a standing position with weight-bearing: (a, c) a.p. radiographs in 20° inner rotation, (b, d) lateral radiographs; (a, b) arthrosis of the upper ankle in the context of rheumatoid arthritis; (c, d) post-traumatic arthrosis with significant supramalleolar valgus malalignment

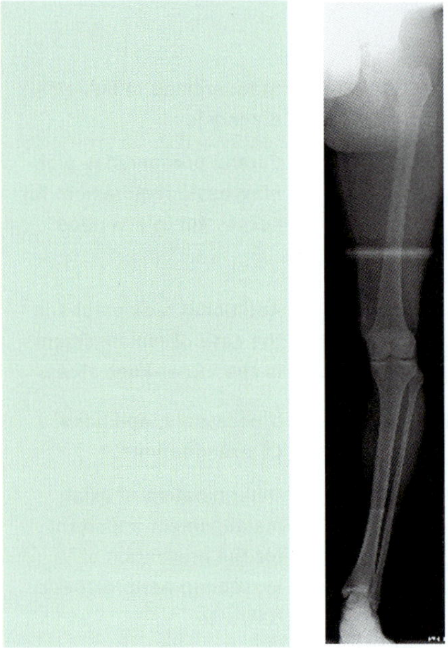

Fig. 4.24: Long leg radiograph on the left in a standing position under weight-bearing, varus malalignment of the knee with secondary valgized hindfoot malalignment.

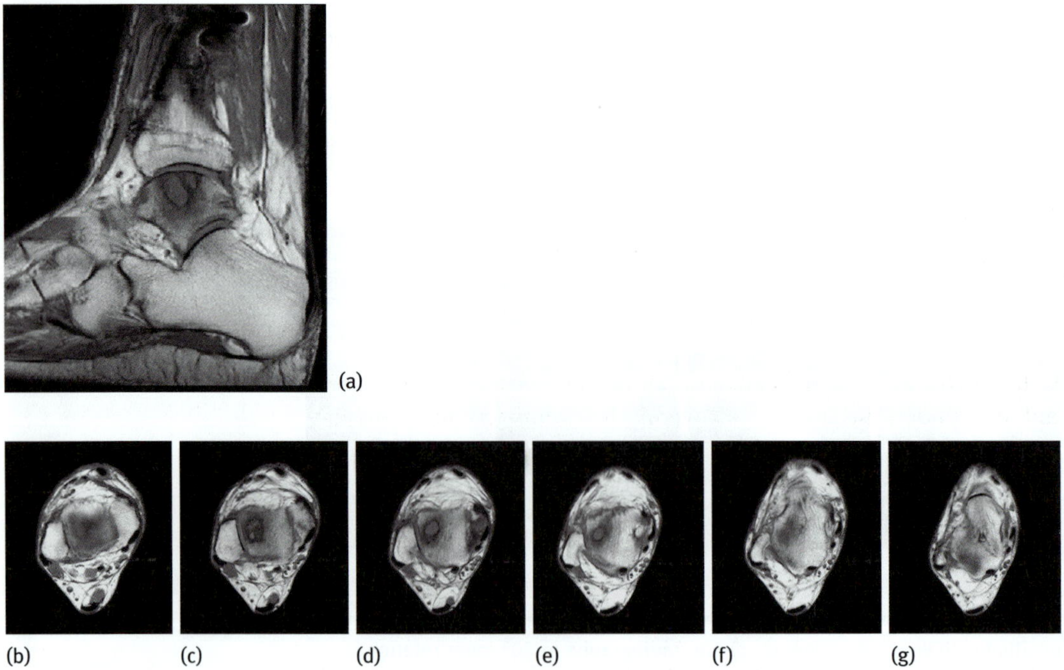

Fig. 4.25: MRT of right ankle (T1) of proximal (a) after distal (g): (a) sagittal layering with depiction of a cyst in the talus, (b–g) transverse depiction of two 0.016 x 0.01 m and 0.003 x 0.003 m cysts in the talus.

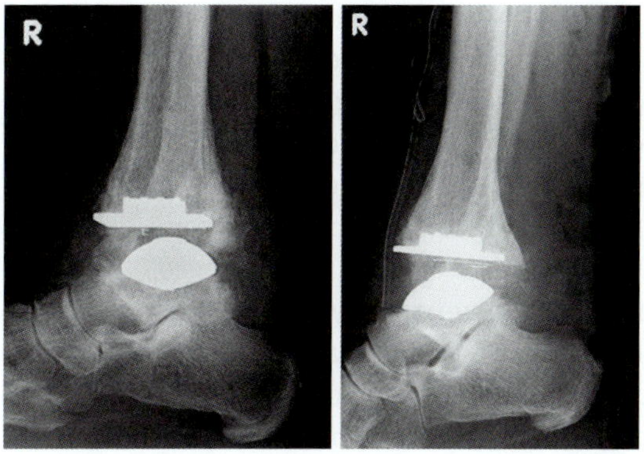

Fig. 4.26: Dorsal and ventral bone impingement eight months after endoprosthesis implantation (S.T.A.R.): (a) preoperative image with significant ossification in the dorsal tibia area with the Achilles tendon affected on movement; (b) postoperative check.

duced in a.p. and lateral projection. Here, too, inner rotation of the ankle of 20° facilitates standardized evaluation.

First follow-up six weeks postoperatively

Six weeks postoperatively the first follow-up after discharge is carried out. To that end the orthotic walker/plaster cast is removed and radiographs are carried out using the aforementioned method. At the point the axial conditions and the bone integration behavior of the prosthesis must be evaluated. Then, full weight-bearing without a orthosis/plaster cast is possible in the case of a normal course.

With a normal course, full weight-bearing without orthosis/plaster cast then possible

X-ray checks after six and twelve months

After six and twelve months, further X-ray checks of secure osseointegration are carried out. Possibly occurring periarticular ossifications with a secondary impingement are noticeable within these periods and can be treated in a timely manner (Fig. 4.26).

4.9 Complications

Possible complications

Complications after endoprosthetic joint replacement of the upper ankle included mechanical problems like impingement and inlay dysfunction, but also fractures and aseptic loosening. Prosthesis infections occur significantly less frequently.

4.9.1 Impingement

Prosthesis impingement: bottleneck phenomenon

Prosthesis impingement can have various causes. Generally speaking, it is a bottleneck phenomenon that leads to local friction and added mechanical stress during joint movement and loading. Bot-

leads to local friction and added mechanical stress during joint movement and loading

tleneck phenomena are usually found in the lateral-medial section (between the medial malleolus and the medial articular facet of the posterior facies articularis talaris), less frequently in the lateral-lateral (lateral malleolus/fibula and the lateral articular facet of the posterior facies articularis talaris) section of the joint of the upper ankle. Ventral and dorsal impingement occurs as a consequence of uncontrolled bone attachment.

Increasing movement- and weight-bearing-dependent pain

Progressive limitation of the initially good joint mobility

Triggers: presumably individual predisposition to the formation of heterotopic bone and mechanical factors

The impingement is characterized by increasing movement- and weight-bearing-dependent pain that can usually be well localized by the patient. Later progressive limitations of the initially good joint mobility may accrue. Friction phenomena occur thereby, both among the bone surfaces and between the prosthesis components and the bone parts. As well as individual predisposition to the formation of heterotopic bone mechanical factors are presumed to be triggers. Initially very narrow and arthrotic, severely destroyed articular facets of the malleolus and the use of talar components that are too large are given equal consideration.

Typical abnormalities in the first one to two years after prosthesis implantation

Diagnostically, not only good anamnestic localization of the pain but also absence of laboratory changes is indicative of the presence of a local impingement syndrome. Radiological findings, such as calcification shadows, osteophytes, and increasing narrowing of the joint space in the area of the articular facets of the malleolus, are among the typical abnormalities that develop one to two years after prosthesis implantation.

Treatment for complaints for 4–8 weeks with the use of intra-articular injection

Statistically growing risk of iatrogenically induced joint infections

Temporary (for 4–8 weeks) the pain and discomfort with the use of intra-articular (diagnostic/therapeutic) injection (local anesthetic with glucocorticoid, e.g., xylocaine 1 % and triamhexal) are usually good for arrest. Depending on the duration of the effect, these injections can be repeated several times. The patient is expressly advised of the statistically growing risk of iatrogenically induced joint infections.

Open arthrolysis with inlay change and removal of calcifications/bone formations in the long term with persistent discomfort and radiological progress

In the long term we carry out in cases of persistent discomfort and radiological progress an open arthrolysis with inlay exchange and removal of calcifications/bone formations. In particular the constrained lateral articular facets are relieved from troublesome bone attachments, in order to create adequate spatial conditions. Usually at this stage the joint surfaces are so destroyed and damaged that adequate spatial conditions without mechanical alteration can only be created after tangential bone resection with the use of oscillating saws. We advise against routine single-shot radiation at the upper ankle with the aim of recidivistic prophylaxis after removal of the ossifications. In our experience, the soft-tissue conditions are very vulnerable here so that after radiation the dreaded wound healing disorders occur significantly more frequently.

4.9.2 Incorrect Sizing of the Prosthesis Parts

As well as the proper positioning of the prosthesis in all three spatial planes, attention is directed to the correct sizing of the prosthesis parts used. The artificial joint replacement is aimed at the most anatomical reconstruction of the joint conditions possible, since only the in this way does the physiological biomechanics of the joint, e.g., the rotation centre and the isometric ligament tension remain preserved. Incorrect sizing of the prosthesis parts can thus change the joint physiology almost as effectively as the malpositioning of the implant.

If components that are too small are chosen, the active pressure loads in the same force and/or weight ratios and reduced surface area must increase under physiological conditions. This can lead to increased wear on the prosthesis (e.g., polyethylene wear, delamination, and aging of the polyethylene), but also to the long-term failure in the area of the prosthesis–bone interface due to aseptic loosening and caving in of the prosthesis.

If the chosen implants are too large they have a suppressive effect locally that has an explosive impact on the anatomically predefined width of the ankle mortise. Oversized tibial components only pass between the malleoli if these are thinned out and/or the syndesmosis is destroyed. In particular, in the area of the medial malleolus the thin, fracture-endangered bone bridge is additionally weakened and thus a "predetermined breaking point" is created. The occurrence of a malleolar fracture can be the consequence immediately at implantation or not until the situation of mobilization with weight-bearing. A talar component that is too big on the other hand works under repetitive weight-bearing (e.g., during walking) like a wedge, that builds up horizontal forces on both malleoli and can trigger stress fractures at the increasingly weakened structure (Fig. 4.27). Additional pressure peaks can arise under weight-bearing in the pronation or supination position of the foot.

Important:
- Proper positioning of the prosthesis on all three spatial planes
- Correct sizing of the prosthesis parts

Prosthesis components that are too small:
- Increased prosthesis wear
- Aseptic loosening and caving in of the prosthesis

Prosthesis components that are too large:
- Suppressive effect with explosive impact on the anatomically predetermined width of the ankle mortise
- Oversized tibial components: malleolar fracture
- Talar components that are too large: stress fractures at the increasingly weakened structure

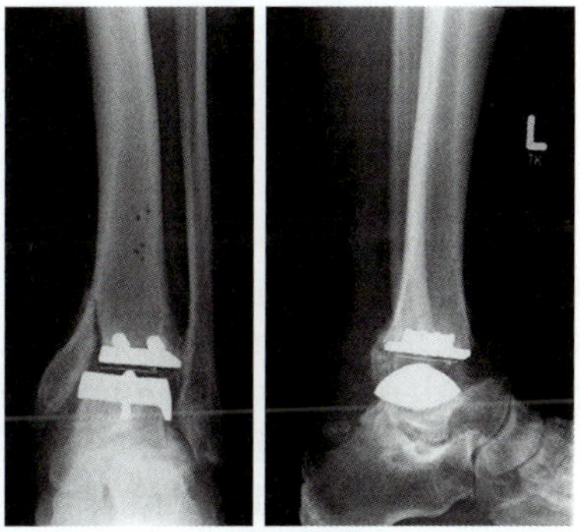

(a) (b)

Fig. 4.27: (a, b) Oversizing of the talar components (S.T.A.R. prosthesis) with consequent stress fracture of the medial malleolus.

4.9.3 Fractures

Fresh malleolar fracture during TEP implantation endangers proper axial alignment of the upper ankle

Preoperative axial deviations high risk of fractures

Malleolar fractures in 6–22 % intraoperatively or shortly after implantation of an upper ankle TEP

Cause: also errors in surgical performance

The proper axial alignment of the upper ankle, especially in the frontal plane, is endangered by the occurrence of fresh malleolar fractures during TEP implantation, which can cause varus and valgus malalignments. Conversely, preoperative axial deviations with or without compromised medial and lateral ligaments represent a high risk of fracture occurring. Breaks in the malleoli happen in 6–22 % of cases intraoperatively or shortly after the implantation of an upper ankle TEP. As well as the aforementioned causes, other errors of surgical performance, such as incorrect placing of the prosthesis, fracture when tapping in the original prosthesis or unduly high traction due to, e.g., bone spreader, are likely causes. Adequate experience and implantation practice thus represent an important preemptive factor in prevention.

Treatment of fractures arising intraoperatively with the use of osteosynthesis

Conservative treatment postoperatively by mobilization of any fractures with the use of lower leg cast/orthosis

Surgical indication: pseudarthrosis formation, persistent pain, axial malalignment

Prophylaxis of postoperative fractures with stabilizing orthoses

Intraoperatively existing fractures should be directly treated with the use of osteosynthesis (screw or tension band osteosynthesis) in the context of the TEP implantation operation. Postoperatively, in the context of fractures occurring during mobilization, low-grade dislocation and axially correct positioning can be treated conservatively with the use of a lower leg cast or orthosis. Here, there is a surgical indication if there is long-term pseudarthrosis formation, persistent pain, and unacceptable axial malalignment. Our patients are mobilized in a stabilizing orthosis (Vacoped®) for four weeks with full weight-bearing for the prophylaxis of postoperative fractures. Depending on the degree of preoperative varus and valgus malalignment, the decision about the surgical possibilities of correction, e.g., lengthening osteotomies of the medial malleolus and/or shortening osteotomy of the lateral malleolus, should be taken in good time. This allows sufficient axial correction with balancing of the medial and lateral ligament, which not least prevents fractures, and helps the (long-term)functioning of the prosthesis to improve significantly.

4.9.4 Aseptic Loosening

Frequency of aseptic loosening 5.4–28 %

Cementless implant fixation recommended

Aseptic loosening of the prosthesis components are among the complications with the highest frequency rate (Fig. 4.28). The data fluctuated wildly between 5.4 and 28 %, depending on the type of prosthesis used and the prevalent type of implant fixation. Essentially, cementless implant fixation has prevailed, and seems to have a favorable effect on the comparably high rates of loosening.

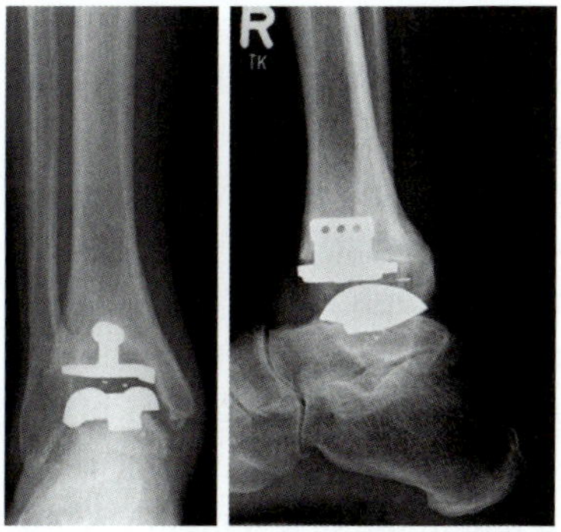

(a) (b)

Fig. 4.28: (a, b) Aseptic loosening with great osteolysis in the area of the medial fixation plug of the tibial component (SALTO prosthesis).

4.9.5 Infections

Infections rare, but dreaded

Infections in the context of ankle endoprosthetics do not have to be included among the most frequent complications, but because of the difficult and long-term course of treatment, the limited treatment alternatives, and the frequent necessity for revision interventions, are among the most dreaded complications.

Revision of 12–20 % of ankle endoprosthesis in 5 years, 9 % because of infection

Approximately 10–20 % of implanted endoprosthesis have to be surgically revised for highly diverse reasons within a follow-up period of five years. Out of these revision operations probably around 9 % are accounted for by infection-induced complications.

Deep wound infections in approximately 1.5–2 %

60–80 % of revisions related to post-traumatic circumstances, joint destruction through chronic polyarthritis

Deep wound infections, i.e., infections with involvement of the implant, must be expected in around 1.5–2 % if implanted upper ankle TEPs. Post-traumatic circumstances and joint destruction in the context of chronic polyarthritis form the most common indication groups. 60–80 % of operations are traced back solely to these two diseases and/or circumstances. Both disease causalities demonstrate a significantly higher risk of infection than in for example primary arthrosis.

4.9.6 Treatment of Prosthesis-Associated Infections of the Upper Ankle

Wound edge necrosis/ wound healing disorders on the basis of peri-/intra-operative errors

Wound edge necroses/wound healing disorders. The origin is often traced back to peri-/intraoperative errors and accordingly for their prevention an experienced implantation and/or surgical technique are sought.

Mechanical loads as low as possible until completion of wound healing

Conditioning of the state of the scars and soft tissue

Lengthening of physiological skin healing through locally impaired wound healing

Healing up of the defects within weeks up to a maximum of 2–3 months

Several treatment options

Until the completion of wound healing the affected patients should be exposed to mechanical loading of the scar that is as low as possible (e.g., through physiotherapy). The main focus is on the conditioning of the state of the scar and soft tissue with the use of immobilization (e.g., orthosis or plaster cast) and detumescent measures (consistent elevation, manual lymph drainage).

Locally impaired wound healing, with or without an area of necrosis of the wound edges, always leads to prolongation of the physiological skin healing beyond the 8th–10th day. At best, these defects heal up within weeks up to a maximum of 2–3 months without consequences. In the case of clinically unremarkable inflammation parameters, regular wound checking/bandage changing, prophylactic antibiotic substitution, and if necessary (surgical) debridement of necrotic tissue, are carried out. The use of vacuum bandages (V.A.C.®), especially in persistent healing disorders, gaping skin defects with or without exposure of the anterior tibia tendon, represent an additional treatment option. They can also be used alternatively for temporary wound coverage up until the wound has definitely closed. Performing open surgical debridement can be equally as indicated in treatment-resistant circumstances as a plastic covering, in order to restore in the long term the state of the closed scars and skin.

Superficial early infections:
- After wound edge necrosis, wound healing disorders
- By perioperatively spread germs

Deep early infections:
- By bacterial contamination during implantation
- On the basis of pre-existing local/generalized infectious states

Early postoperative infections. Early infections occur within the first 4–6 weeks after the operation/prosthesis implantation and are divided into superficial and deep infections. Superficial early infections can arise secondarily at the base of the wound edge necrosis and/or wound healing disorders (see above) or primarily through germs spread perioperatively. Deep early infections are rarities and arise through bacterial contamination during prosthesis implantation or at the base of pre-existing local/generalized infectious states. The routine prophylaxis with the use of systemically and locally applied antibiotics constitutes the most vital protection from an early infection.

Early infections often with typical onset and course

Frequent symptoms

The clinical follow-up straight after the operation is important because early infections often demonstrate a typical onset and course. Severe wound pain immediately postoperatively, which lasts unusually long (over several days) and above-average requests for analgesic doses by the affected patient, are often observed as locally florid and swollen wound conditions. Gaping wound edges and/or inflamed wound edge discoloration may occur as well as increased wound secretion. Clinically, the initially high CRP values remain static for the rest of the course (>100 mg/l) or increase again.

The treatment of early infection can essentially be carried out both for superficial and deep infections with preservation of the ankle prosthesis. Among the treatment options for superficial early infection are debridement, thorough rinsing, and possibly the sparing resection of the wound edges. Complete wound closure is attempted in every case and can if necessary be achieved with the use of a plastic cover. Vacuum sealing bandages represent a temporary alternative to reducing the defect and to stimulating the formation of granulation tissue. Postoperatively, antibiotics are administered for 6–12 weeks (beginning systemically and later continued orally), which if possible must be adapted to the availability of the antiobiogram. Continuous (2–3 days) monitoring of the laboratory inflammation parameters is carried out for this period.

Treatment of early infection with preservation of the ankle prosthesis

Complete wound closure attempted

6–12 weeks antibiotics administration postoperatively

Continuous monitoring of the inflammation parameters

Deep infections are treated according to a similar schedule. The surgical procedures are carried out, considering the greater spread of infection, with penetration of the retinaculum and attack of the prosthesis, more extensively and more invasively. The debridement and synovectomy must certainly involve the dorsal joint and capsule areas, which is why it is obligatory to exchange the polyethylene inlay. With the right indications and an interval of six weeks at the most (but four weeks is better) after primary TEP implantation, around 60–80 % of cases can be successfully treated in this way.

Treatment of deep infections according to a similar schedule

Successful treatment for the right indications and short interval after primary TEP implantation in 60–80 % of cases

Low-grade infections. The long disease course of low-grade infections is usually accompanied by unapparent and non-specific symptoms and typically results in prosthesis loosening. Microbiological detection of bacteria often does not succeed. *Staphylococcus epidermidis* is diagnosed as the most common pathogen by far. In the case of persistent diagnostic uncertainty (distinction: aseptic loosening vs. low-grade infection), antibiotics treatment lasting several weeks can be tried. However, if the induced diagnosis and/or treatment remains unsuccessful, surgical exploration should be contemplated as the remaining option.

Low-grade infections with long disease course and prosthesis loosening

Microbiological detection of bacteria rare

- Antibiotics treatment lasting several weeks
- Surgical exploration as the last option

In our view, the frequency of low-grade infections is significantly underestimated. Proven low-grade infections, as well as all uncertain cases, constitute a clear indication for a two-stage prosthesis revision.

Proven low-grade infections indication for two-stage prosthesis change

Deep late infection. Late infections can appear at any time during the entire life time of the patient, especially after primarily successful prosthesis infection, and show a broad palette of triggering pathogens.

Late infections possible at any time during a lifetime

Two-stage prosthesis revision method of choice

The two-stage prosthesis revision is also the method of choice in these cases. Whether after successful infection treatment a permanent arthrodesis can be carried out still remains an individual decision that among other things is taken jointly with the patient after intensive explanation.

4.9.7 Postoperative Movement Limitations

Preoperative movement determines the functional result after upper ankle implantation

Treatment of postoperative movement limitations conservatively or with surgical procedures

The functional result after implantation of a total endoprosthesis at the upper ankle is, apart from a correct execution of the operation, essentially co-determined by preoperative mobility. In particular, post-traumatic upper ankle arthrodesis often has a tendency toward pronounced movement limitations preoperatively, which can be improved by the operation in only a limited way. The ability of dorsal extension is usually particularly affected by the functional deficits. This has a sustained effect on the heel-to-toe roll and the healthy gait physiology. But progressive ossification/heterotopic bone formation, impingement problems with increasing movement limitation, and implant malpositioning are also possible triggers. Depending on the causal genesis, after exhausting the conservative possibilities (movement exercises, gait training, stretching exercises, midfoot rockers), surgical procedures such as prosthesis revisions, Achilles tendon lengthening, and open arthrolysis with removal of ossifications are considered.

4.10 After Care

No uniform after care regime

There is no uniform after care regime. The various concepts range from immediate postoperative full weight-bearing up to non-weight-bearing for several weeks. Likewise, a plaster cast or orthotic treatment does not have to be standard.

After care program of the Orthopedic University Clinic of Magdeburg

In the following, the after care program of the Orthopedic University Clinic of Magdeburg is presented (Tab. 4.2).

Table 4.2: Rehabilitation program after ankle endoprosthesis (Orthopedic University Clinic of Magdeburg).

Phase I: After removal of the circular lower leg walking cast	
Aims	– Pain reduction – Swelling reduction – Recovery of movement – Protection from re-injury
Therapeutic exercises/ protection measures	– Use of under arm crutches until recovery of a fluid gait, if necessary, taping – Ice, if needed cold-hot packs, Kryocuff, ice machine or ice pack as well as cold air, light compression with elastic wrap or orthosis – Keeping raised, raised above heart level – Manual lymph drainage as needed – Active movement exercises – Manual therapy for the forefoot – Gait training
Phase II: Mobilization phase	
Aims	– Pain reduction – Increase in painless range of movement – Beginning of strengthening – Beginning of non-weight-bearing, proprioceptive training – Reduction of the necessary support – Removal of the measures to reduce pain and swelling: ice, bathes, ultrasound (not in the area of the prosthesis); manual lymph drainage – Weight-bearing: increase in the load up to full body weight under gait training conditions
Therapeutic exercises	– Active range of movement exercise, dorsal flexion, inversion, foot circle plantar flexion, eversion, foot alphabet – Exercise to improve strength: isometric exercise in pain-free area, raising two dumbbells with hand towel, picking up objects with the toes – Proprioceptive training: if possible, exercise on the balance board – tretching: passive range of movement, only dorsal flexion/plantar flexion in the pain-free area, no passive, non-controlled eversion and inversion, Achilles stretching – Joint mobilization in the forefoot area
Phase III: Early rehabilitation phase	
Aims	– Increase in the range of movement – Further progress in strengthening of the proprioceptive training, painless activities of daily life, painless full weight-bearing – Normal gait pattern
Therapeutic exercises	– Stretching of the gastrocnemius and soleus with increasing intensity, joint mobilization in the forefoot and midfoot areas – Strengthening: increasing weights with use of heels, toes, steps, small side lunges, eccentric, concentric exercises (Theraband); no eversion and inversion (prevention of ankle impingement); plantar flexion, dorsal flexion, peroneal strengthening, and isokinetics – If possible, proprioceptive training (proceeding form partial weight-bearing to full weight-bearing): standing on the wobble board, carefully beginning balancing on one leg, continuing therapy if there is any pain and swelling still present with support tape

Table 4.2: (Continued)

Phase IV: Return to every-day and working life intensity	
Aims	– Achievement of full weight-bearing, nearing normal biomechanical conditions – Protection from overstraining the joint and instability
Therapeutic exercises	– Continuation of strengthening exercise and range of movement – Terrain training – Exercises in fast walking, varying walking loads with softer and harder padding – Exercises in the flowing water channel without fins – PNF techniques, Janda's short foot – Treadmill therapy – Accompanying therapy of achieving general fitness: upper body ergometer, bicycle ergometer, stomach/back exercises, strengthening exercise for the healthy leg

4.10.1 In the Clinic

Weight-adapted thrombosis prophylaxis

Weight-adapted thrombosis prophylaxis with low-molecular-weight heparin and compression stockings is standard. New oral direct Factor Xa inhibitors are currently undergoing licensing and will certainly play a large role in clinical and outpatient routine in the future.

Compression bandage padded with absorbent cotton to prevent lymphedema

Positioning of the leg on a Braun's splint

Club foot prophylaxis

While in the operating room the patients receive a compression bandage padded with absorbent cotton. This has proved successful in the context of the prevention of lymphedema and is reapplied by the physiotherapist after each successive treatment. The positioning of the leg on a Braun's splint is also recommended. For club foot prophylaxis an additional pad is used (Fig. 4.29). According to the contents, the drain that has been inserted should be removed on the second/third postoperative day.

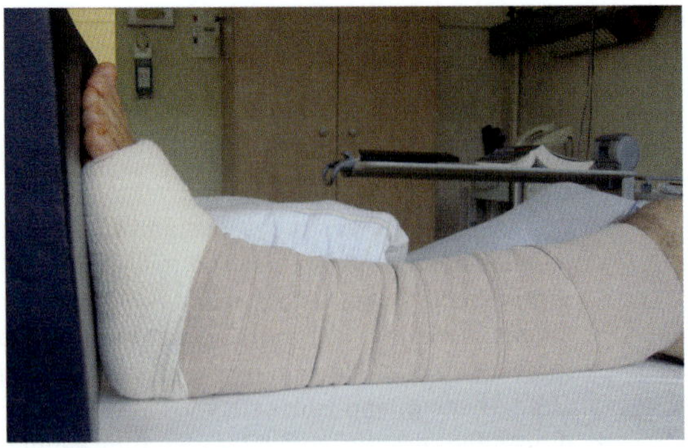

Fig. 4.29: Postoperative positioning in bed. Club foot prophylaxis is carried out with the use of a prepositioned pad at the end of the foot. The patients must be intensively educated about the necessity of this sometimes painful method.

Table 4.3: Example of a pain therapy schedule after ankle endoprosthesis.

	Day 0 day of op.	Postop. day 1	Postop. day 2	Postop. day 3	Postop. day 4	Postop. day 5	Postop. day 6	Postop. day 7	Postop. day 8	Postop. day 9	Postop. day 10
PDK placement/day	3–4×	3–4×	3–4×	3–4×	PDK removal	–	–	–	–	–	–
Metamizole	3–4× 1 g p.o.	3–4× 1 g p.o.	3–4× 1 g p.o.	3–4× 1 g p.o.	3–4× 1 g p.o.	3–4× 1 g p.o.	3–4× 1 g p.o.	3–4× 1 g p.o.	–	–	–
Etoricoxib	1× 90–120 mg p.o.	1× 90–120 mg p.o.	1× 90–120 mg p.o.	1× 90–120 mg p.o.	1× 90–120 mg p.o.	1× 90–120 mg p.o.	1× 90–120 mg p.o.	1× 90–120 mg p.o.	1× 90–120 mg p.o.	1× 90–120 mg p.o.	1× 90–120 mg p.o.
Esmeprazole	1× 40 mg p.o. at night	1× 40 mg p.o. at night	1× 40 mg p.o. at night	1× 40 mg p.o. at night	1× 40 mg p.o. at night	1× 40 mg p.o. at night	1× 40 mg p.o. at night	1× 40 mg p.o. at night	1× 40 mg p.o. at night	1× 40 mg p.o. at night	1× 40 mg p.o. at night
Additional piritramide as needed	Up to 4× 15 mg s.c.	Up to 4× 15 mg s.c.	Up to 4× 15 mg s.c.	Up to 4× 15 mg s.c.	–	–	–	–	–	–	–

Analgesia. Operations on the ankle can be carried out under general or local anesthetic or in combination of both procedures. Most patients in our clinic are operated on under regional anesthesia (spinal anesthesia) in combination with a peridural catheter for postoperative analgesia. Regional anesthesia procedures are usually combined with the use of hypnosis or a sedative, which leads to significantly higher patient acceptance.

General or regional anesthesia or a combination of both procedures

The possibility of maintenance injections via the peridural catheter is deployed in postoperative analgesia management. In the context of physiotherapeutic exercising, the catheter can be loaded intermittently with use of single doses or continuously via a perfusor. Single doses should be administered approximately 30 minutes before the physiotherapeutic exercise. In this way, pain-free exercise is possible in most cases.

Postoperative analgesia management with maintenance injections via the peridural catheter

For oral medication the usual peripherally effective analgesics are used. In patients with a known predisposition for heterotopic ossifications a prophylaxis with non-steroidal anti-inflammatory drugs (NSAIDs) should be carried out.

The usual peripherally effective analgesics for oral medication

A pain therapy schedule used at the Orthopedic University Clinic of Magdeburg is shown in Tab. 4.3.

Pain therapy schedule

In our view, gastric protection should then be carried out, if no NSAIDs are used, since the general stress of the operation alone can constitute a gastric risk.

Gastric protection recommended

Physiotherapy. On the day of the operation the pain therapy is the top priority and physiotherapeutic exercise should not be carried out. However, club foot prophylaxis with the use of splint positioning should take place immediately (Fig. 4.29).

Operation day: pain therapy

Club foot prophylaxis with use of splint positioning

If possible from the 1st postoperative day lymph drainage for the lower leg

Via the ventral surgical approach, the deriving lymph nodes can be affected. Lymph drainage disorders with fore- and midfoot swelling are not rare and require more attention from the physiotherapist. If the condition of all the wounds allows it, lymph drainage for the whole lower leg is prescribed from the 1st postoperative day, in order to prevent edema. To increase the patient's tolerance adequate analgesic treatment should be observed.

Adequate analgesic treatment

Passive physiotherapeutic exercise treatments from the 1st postoperative day

Furthermore, from the 1st postoperative day we begin with passive physiotherapeutic exercise treatments. Above all, these serve to prevent adhesions in the area of the paratenon of the extensor under the retinaculum and the Achilles tendon. In cases of preexisting movement limitations constructive mobilization techniques such as the post-isometric relaxation (PIR) may be used. Also, manual stretching of the triceps surae is vital in the early phase. Here, particular attention must be paid after percutaneous Achilles tenotomy, since the intraoperative range of movement (especially dorsal extension)can only be preserved by intensive training. For many patients in whom movement has been limited for several years, this represents a particular problem and must thus be supported by adequate pain therapy.

Support with adequate pain therapy

Active exercise during the following days

According to the compliance of the patient they can go straight on to active supported and/or active exercise during the following days. Pronation and supination should be avoided. After each treatment the compression bandage is reapplied.

Walker orthosis on the 8th postoperative day

Provided there is uncomplicated wound healing, on the 8th postoperative day we get the patient on a walker orthosis (e.g., VACO®ped orthosis). With this, full weight-bearing on under arm crutches is normally possible. Follow-up gait training and learning to walk on stairs ensure that the patient settles back into their home environment.

Gait training and learning to walk on stairs

Plaster cast necessary in rare cases

In rare cases a plaster cast is necessary. This often affects patients for whom shoes cannot be provided because of their size. As the orthosis must be worn day and night, patients with low compliance are also provided with a circular lower leg cast/plaster. This also used in the context of follow-up care after intraoperative malleolar fractures or simultaneous conversion osteotomies.

Removal of the suture material, discharge on 10th postoperative day

In our clinic we try to exercise patients 2–3 times daily after ankle endoprosthesis. On the 10th postoperative day the suture material is removed and the patient discharged to further outpatient treatment.

4.10.2 Outpatients

After discharge the osseointegration of the endoprosthesis is the top priority. The orthosis should usually continue to be worn for a further four weeks after discharge (day and night). A removable sole on the walker orthosis helps to maintain a minimum of level of hygiene. It can be removed after entering the home. Because uncontrolled movements must be expected during sleep, the orthosis should not be removed at nighttime.

Osseointegration of the endoprosthesis

Continuous wearing of the orthosis for a further four weeks after discharge

The use of crutches can be progressively reduced. First, they can be dispensed with at home. When walking longer distances the underarm crutches should be used for four weeks postoperatively. This can be managed more leniently in patients with a high level of compliance.

Progressive reduction in the use of crutches

Six weeks after the operation, an X-ray examination should be carried out. In the case of an uneventful course with axially correct alignment and no signs of loosening the orthosis can be removed. The patients should initially wear a high, closed custom-made shoe. If there is no discomfort a free choice of shoes is possible. High-heeled shoes should only be worn occ asionally and reserved for certain days.

X-ray check six weeks postoperatively

In the case of an uneventful course removal of the orthosis

Free choice of shoes if no discomfort

Analgesia. After discharge to further outpatient care the patients are usually mobilized on two underarm crutches in the walker orthosis or in a cast. Normally they need only few or no analgesics at this time. Continuation of the medications prescribed at discharge is recommended. They can be slowly tapered over the course of the next two weeks.

After discharge few or no analgesics necessary

After removal of the orthosis/cast, physiotherapeutic exercise is applied. Here, renewed analgesic support should be effected, especially at the start.

If necessary analgesia for physiotherapeutic exercise

4.10.3 Rehabilitation Measures

After removal of the orthosis/cast, intensive physiotherapeutic exercise must be carried out. A stationary, semi-stationary or ambulant rehabilitation measure is recommended. Stationary measures occasionally lead to problems with medical insurance since discharge from the hospital is usually too long ago. It is easier for patients to organize within the scope of occupational therapy.

Stationary, semi-stationary or ambulant rehabilitation measures recommended

A minimum amount of exercise, at least through adequate physiotherapy, must be carried out however. Gait training with coordination exercise, terrain and ADL training (ADL = activities of daily living) are required, especially in patients who are still in

Minimum of exercise through adequate physiotherapy

employment, in order to enable a return to everyday loading situations as quickly as possible. Electrotherapy, cold therapy, and water training constitute an ideal extension of the measures mentioned.

80 % of the expected range of movement up to five months after the operation

Because up to five months after the operation 80 % of the expected range of movement is achieved, as far as possible during this time the prescription of standardized drug combinations is continued.

References

Beaudoin AJ, Fiore SM, Krause WR, Adelaar RS. Effect of isolated talocalcaneal fusion on contact in the ankle and talonavicular joints. Foot Ankle 1991;12(1):19–25.

Conti SF, WongYS. Complications of total ankle replacement. Clin Orthop Relat Res 2001;391:105–14.

Doets HC, van der Plaat LW, Klein JP. Medial malleolar osteotomy for the correction of varus deformity during total ankle arthroplasty: results in 15 ankles. Foot Ankle Int 2008;29(2):171–7.

Doets HC, van Middelkoop M, Houdijk H, Nelissen RG, et al. Gait analysis after successful mobile bearing total ankle replacement. Foot Ankle Int 2007;28(3):313–22.

Eichinger S, Forst R, Kindervater M. Indications and alternatives for arthroplasty in young patients. Orthopade 2007;36(4):311–24.

Endres T, Grass R, Rammelt S, Zwipp H. Ankle arthrodesis with four cancellous lag screws. Oper Orthop Traumatol 2005;17(4–5):345–60.

Fevang BT, Lie SA, Havelin LI, Brun JG, et al. 257 ankle arthroplastiesperformed in Norway between 1994 and 2005. Acta Orthop 2007;78(5):575–83.

Geipel U, Herrmann M. The infected implant: bacteriology. Unfallchirurg 2005;108(11):961–75; quiz 976–7.

Gould JS, Alvine FG, Mann RA, Sanders RW, et al. Total ankle replacement: a surgical discussion. Part II. The clinical and surgical experience. Am J Orthop 2000;29(9):675–82.

Grass R, Rammelt S, Biewener A, Zwipp H. Arthrodesis of the ankle joint. Clin Podiatr Med Surg 2004;21(2):161–78.

Grass R, Rammelt S, Endres T, Zwipp H. Reorientational arthrodesis of the ankle joint using four screws. Orthopade 2005;34(12):1209–15.

Haddad SL, Coetzee JC, Estok R, Fahrbach K, et al. Intermediate and longterm outcomes of total ankle arthroplasty and ankle arthrodesis. A systematic review of the literature. J Bone Joint Surg Am 2007;89(9):1899–905.

Hamblen DL. Can the ankle joint be replaced? J Bone Joint Surg Br 1985;67(5):689–90.

Hamel J. Anterior tibial tendon transfer in ankle replacement – early experience. Fuß & Sprunggelenk 2008;6:37–44.

Haskell A, Mann RA. Ankle arthroplasty with preoperative coronal plane deformity: short-term results. Clin Orthop Relat Res 2004;424:98–103.

Havelin LI, Engesaeter LB, Espehaug B, Furnes O, et al. The Norwegian Arthroplasty Register:11 years and 73,000 arthroplasties. Acta Orthop Scand 2000;71(4):337–53.

Henricson A, Skoog A, Carlsson A. The Swedish Ankle Arthroplasty Register: An analysis of 531 arthroplasties between 1993 and 2005. Acta Orthop 2007;78(5):569–74.
Hintermann B, Knupp M, Barg A. Osteotomies of the distal tibia and hindfoot for ankle realignment. Orthopaede 2005;37(3):212–8, 220–3.
Hintermann B, Valderrabano V. Total ankle replacement. Foot Ankle Clin 2003;8(2):375–405.
Kakkar AK, Brenner B, Dahl OE, Eriksson BI, et al. Extended duration rivaroxaban versus short-term enoxaparin for the prevention of venous thromboembolism after total hip arthroplasty: a double-blind, randomized controlled trial. Lancet 2008;372(9632):31–9.
Kofoed H, Lundberg-Jensen A. Ankle arthroplasty in patients younger and older than 50 years: a prospective series with long-term follow-up. Foot Ankle Int 1999;20(8):501–6.
Lidgren L. Joint prosthetic infections: a success story. Acta Orthop Scand 2001;72(6):553–6.
Lord G, Marotte JH. Total ankle prosthesis. Technic and 1st results. Apropos of 12 cases. Rev Chir Orthop Reparatrice Appar Mot 1973;59(2):139–51.
Lord G, Marotte JH. Total ankle replacement (author's transl). Rev Chir Orthop Reparatrice Appar Mot 1980;66(8):527–30.
Myerson M. Reconstructive Foot and Ankle Surgery 2005. Philadelphia: Elsevier Saunders, 2005:500.
Neumann HW, Lieske S, Schenk K. Supramalleolar, subtractive valgus osteotomy of the tibia in the management of ankle joint degeneration with varus deformity. Oper Orthop Traumatol 2007;19(5–6):511–26.

M. Nottrott, A. Streitbürger, S. Höll, G. Gosheger, J. Hardes

5 Tumor Endoprosthetics

5.1 Indications

At the beginning of the era of tumor endoprostheses an individually produced special implant was used in each case. However, this brought with it serious disadvantages. On the one hand, the production was very expensive; on the other it was also time-consuming. Manufacture usually lasted around six weeks; thus, to some extent, the optimal operative time for the resection of the tumor could not be adhered to and so the whole prognosis of the patient was significantly impeded. Another disadvantage was the lack of possibility of intraoperative variation after completion of the implant. Not infrequently, the exact size or, for example, the stem diameter turned out to be different from what was planned beforehand from the X-ray, but the possibility of changing or adapting the implant was non-existent. This led to somewhat worse functioning and premature failure of the prosthesis.

Tumor endoprostheses individually produced special implants to start with

- Production expensive, time-consuming

- Lacking possibility of intraoperative variation

To satisfy the patient and surgeon, new implants were therefore necessary, which were available without intensive preoperative planning at justifiable cost within the shortest time, offered a wide range of possibilities of intraoperative variation, and thus enabled adaptation to each individual anatomical situation. The modern modular tumor prosthesis systems fulfill these requirements. The modularity makes it possible to individually reconstruct bone defects in any size, without having to make compromises in stability and durability. Although young and physically very active patients are usually affected, who make extreme demands on the material and fixation, in the last 30 years the 5-year survival rate of megaendoprostheses has risen significantly from around 20 % to 85 %.

Modern modular tumor prosthesis systems:

- Justifiable costs
- Available in the shortest time
- Wide range of possibilities of intraoperative variation

5-year survival rate of megaendoprostheses at 85 %

The classic indication for tumor prostheses is an extensive bone defect after further resection of a malignant primary bone tumor of the meta-diaphyseal region, usually at the lower extremity. Tumor prostheses, however, are also used in solitary bone metastases of special primary tumors (e.g., renal cell carcinoma) or in the reconstruction of non-tumor-induced bone defects, as they may exist after fractures or after explantation of an infected prosthesis (Fig. 5.1). In revision endoprosthetics so-called tumor prostheses also have increased application. Nowadays, many previous contraindications to prosthesis implantation have to be reconsidered.

Indications:

- Extensive bone defect after bone tumor resection
- Solitary bone metastases
- Reconstruction of non-tumor-induced bone defects
- Revision endoprosthetics

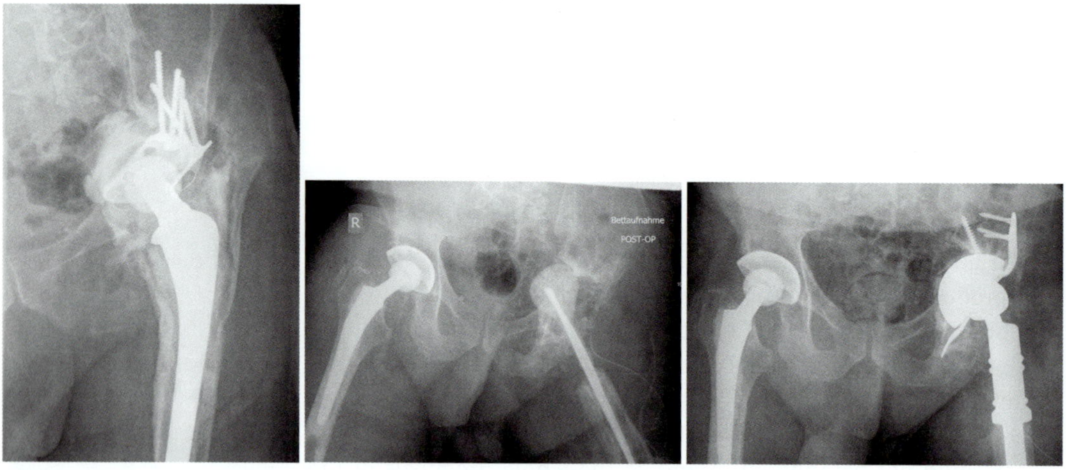

(a) (b) (c)

Fig. 5.1: Infected left-sided hip endoprosthesis (a), two-stage revision with explantation of the infected prosthesis and spacer implantation (b) as well as reconstruction of the proximal femur with a Mutars® proximal femur prosthesis after infection removal.

5.2 Preoperative Planning

Precise preoperative planning essential requirement

Precise planning of the implant with Auto-CAD software and digital templates

The exact preoperative planning is an essential component of the implantation of a tumor prosthesis. Today, the section of the extremity affected is digitally X-rayed in a standardized manner with a measuring rod at bone level in order to be able to compensate for the radiological enlargement factors for planning purposes. Afterward, the implant can be precisely planned using Auto-CAD software and digital templates. This preoperative planning shows whether the implantation of standardized modular prosthesis components are possible or maybe custom-made product must be made to solve the problem. On the basis of the intraoperatively representative finding, which, despite careful preoperative preparation, can deviate from the plan, the surgeon must finally decide intraoperatively which prosthesis components should be implanted. In over 90 % of cases of our own group, however, the preoperative planning could be put into practice.

5.3 Current Tumor Endoprosthesis Systems

Various modular tumor prosthesis systems available

In the meantime, several modular tumor prosthesis systems from various manufacturers are on the market, that in general are all very similar, but partly exhibit significant differences. What all systems have in common is a modular construction, usually consisting of cemented or cementlessly implanted stems, which are then connected to the corresponding modular replacement of the resected

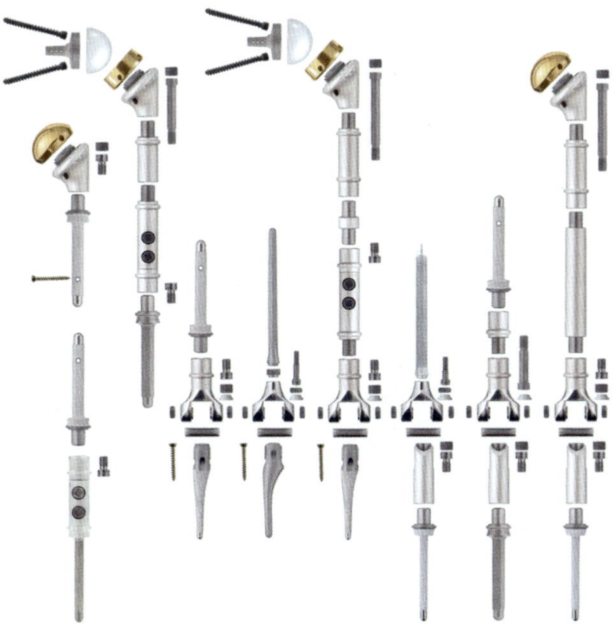

Fig. 5.2: Overview of modular tumor endoprosthesis components of Mutars® Silver System for the reconstruction of the upper extremity.

bone and the joint mechanism. At the upper extremity, reconstruction of the proximal humerus, the humeral diaphysis, the distal humerus, the proximal ulna, as well as the replacement of the whole humerus is possible (Fig. 5.2).

Reconstructions at the upper extremity

At the lower extremity, reconstruction of the proximal femur, the femoral diaphysis, the distal femur, the whole femur, the proximal tibia, the tibial diaphysis as well as the distal tibia and the whole tibia with custom-made products is possible (Fig. 5.3).

Reconstructions at the lower extremity

With regard to the possibilities of soft-tissue reconstruction, however, there are great differences. The GMRS™ (Global Modular Replacement System) from Stryker® provides the prostheses for example with special surfaces and/or loops that are supposed to guarantee adherence of the ligaments to the metal. To some extent, a combination of the prosthesis with an allograft is also carried out, which then serves as refixation of the soft-tissue structures. On the basis of the significantly increased danger of infection linked with this, however, allografts are used in Germany with great reluctance.

Soft-tissue reconstruction with very different systems

The standard tumor prosthesis system used is the "Modular Universal Tumor and Revision System" (Mutars®) by Implantcast® (Buxtehude). The modular design has been in use since 1992 and was developed at the University Clinic Münster. Because of its modular-

Modular Universal Tumor and Revision System (Mutars®)

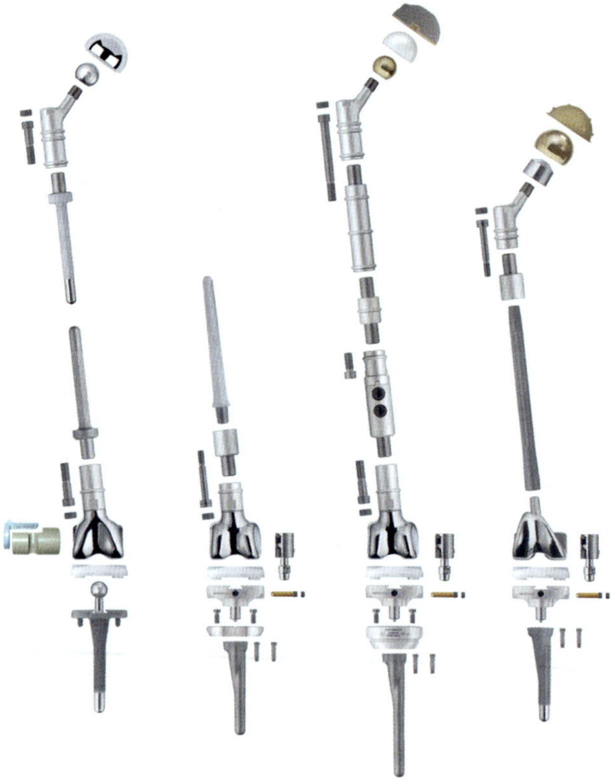

Fig. 5.3: Overview of modular tumor endoprosthesis components of Mutars® Silver System for the reconstruction of the lower extremity

▸ Individual reconstruction

▸ Cemented or cementless stem fixation

▸ Hydroxyapatite-coated titanium stem

▸ Cemented fixation in the elderly, osteoporosis, chemotherapy

ity, this system allows individual reconstruction of bone defects of any size, not only after tumor resections, but also after fractures or removal of infected implants.

The bone fixation of the prosthesis stem is done with or without cement. On the basis of the hexagonal cross-section (Fig. 5.4) secure stem fixation with excellent primary rotation stability of 70 nm (median) is possible. The stem design for the distal femur achieves additional stability through consideration of the physiological antecurvature. After drilling of the bone, suitably preformed hexagonal rasps guarantee an exact fit and secure press-fit fixation.

For cementless fixation the Mutars® system uses hydroxyapatite coasted titanium stems (titanium alloy $TiAl_6V_4$), whose most common stem length is 0.12 m. The diameter is individually planned with the aid of digital radiography, but should not if possible fall below a core diameter of 0.012 m because of the stability required. A cemented fixation (CoCr casting alloy) is usually necessary in older patients (over 60 years) and/or in cases of osteoporo-

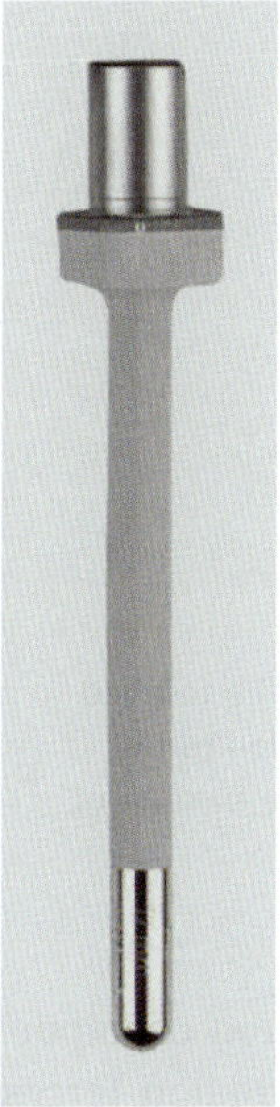

Fig. 5.4: Cementless, hexagonal, hydroxyapatite-coated stem of the Mutars® System.

sis, e.g., due to long preoperative immobilization and/or neoadjuvant chemotherapy; it is however also recommended if a press-fit fixation in the meta-diaphyseal region is not possible.

Toothed connecting face for prevention/correction of rotational errors

All prosthesis modules are held at their points of attachment with a toothed connecting face, by which the rotation can be very precisely adjusted in 5° increments even after firm fixation of the stems (Fig. 5.5). Through this system rotational errors can be prevented and, if necessary, corrected. To restore the length of bone removed, extension pieces are available in 1 to 2 cm increments. These are also supplied with a toothed connecting face. After correct adjustment and checking of rotation with the joint component they are connected to the stem and fixed with screws.

Endoprosthetic replacement including the knee joint:
- Rotational knee joint and PEEK Optima® locking device
- Metal-on-metal locking device

An endoprosthetic replacement including the knee joint requires an extraordinary combination of flexibility and stability, in particular because the cruciate as well as the collateral ligaments also have to be resected. The joint replacement consists of a constrained rotational knee joint ("rotating hinge") and the PEEK Optima® locking device, which demonstrates significantly greater stability. The Metal-on-Metal (MOM) locking device is a further development that connects the femoral component and tibial component via a metal pin and thus improves the durability by far. The insertion of a "rotating hinge" allows flexion of up to around 95° and extension as well as a certain degree of rotation with simultaneous stabilization in cases of varus/valgus stress and move-

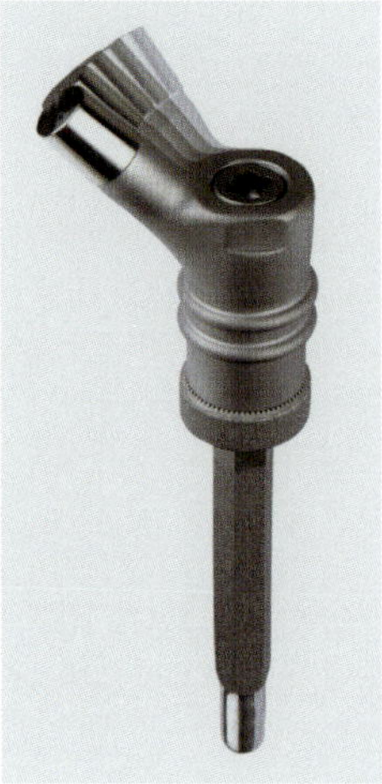

Fig. 5.5: Mutars® proximal femur. The toothed connecting face also enables rotation to be adjusted in 5° increments after firm fixation of the stem.

ments in the anterior–posterior plane. This preservation of important movement abilities reduces the transfer of the torsion forces to the stem fixation and joint mechanisms, thus reducing the rate of loosening and wear of the polyethylene parts. Soft-tissue reconstruction and the secure refixation of tendons and muscles succeeds through the use of a Mutars® attachment tube made of *polyethylene terephthalate, as described in section 9.6.1 "Soft Tissue Reconstruction."*

▸ Reduction in loosening rate and wear of the PE parts

In intra-articular proximal femur resections the hip joint is typically reconstructed with a proximal femur replacement in combination with a dual head. If a reconstruction of the acetabulum in an existing arthrosis should be necessary, an "antiluxation socket" in the form of a tripolar socket (e.g., Avantage socket from Biomet) constitutes an alternative that also prevents postoperative luxation in a poor soft tissue situation.

Antiluxation socket in reconstruction of the acetabulum prevents postoperative luxation

In resections of the proximal humerus and the subsequent reconstruction, the functional result is directly dependent on the preservation of the nervus axillaris and the rotator cuff. As the tumor resections are often accompanied by a loss in particular of the nerve, in order to create an adequate safety margin with the tumor, patients cannot perform basic abduction and elevation of the arm. In contrast, in benign tumors, metastases, low-grade tumors, or in prosthesis revisions, the preservation of the nervus axillaris is often possible; thus, inverse proximal humeral prostheses can be applied. These demonstrate a better functional result, since, analogous to the inverse shoulder endoprosthetics, in rotator cuff insufficiencies, the medialization of the center of rotation compensates for the (partially) resected rotator cuff and thereby cause a stronger control of the musculus deltoideus.

Functional result in resection and reconstruction of the proximal humerus dependent on the preservation of the nervus axillaris and rotator cuff

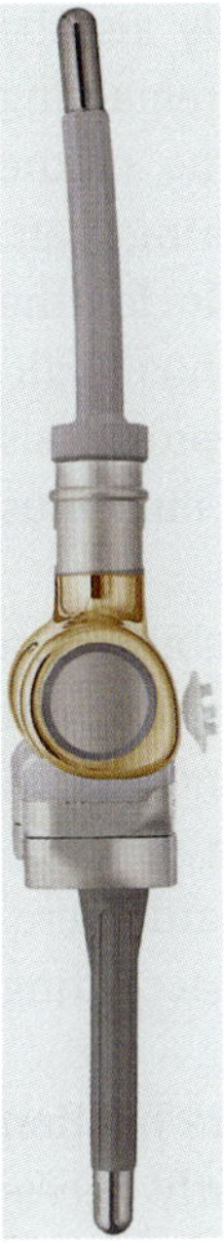

Fig. 5.6: Silver-coated Mutars® prosthesis: distal femur to reduce periprosthetic infection.

For special indications, separate prosthesis coatings are available. For the prevention of allergic reactions a titanium nitrite coating is available in the case of such a suspicion. On the basis of the great danger of infection of the megaendoprostheses a special antibacterial silver coating (Mutars® Silver) was developed, which seemed to be responsible for a significant reduction in the infection rates, so far without relevant side effects (Fig. 5.6). Despite the numerous variations possible, if custom-made products or special adapters should be necessary for combining with other prosthesis systems, these have become available in a relatively short time from the prosthesis company (Implantcast®).

Separate prosthesis coatings for special indications

- Antibacterial silver coating reduces infection rates
- Custom-made products or special adapters available

5.3.1 Soft Tissue Reconstruction

The functional result of a tumor prosthesis is directly dependent on the functional soft tissues and muscles that are still available after resection. The basic aims of the soft-tissue reconstruction are on the one hand, the tension-free coverage of the prosthesis and on the other, the restoration of muscular function and stability. Here, the indication for a muscle flap graft (above all at the proximal tibia) should be liberally provided, as complete coverage of the prosthesis in muscle minimizes the great danger of wound necrosis and infections. In order to achieve adequate resection

Soft-tissue reconstruction:
- Tension-free coverage of the prosthesis
- Restoration of muscular function and stability
- Application of a muscle flap graft

margins, portions of the quadriceps muscle must usually also be removed in tumor resections in of the distal femur. If the remaining musculature does not guarantee satisfactory functioning of the joint, parts of the quadriceps can be replaced by a hamstring graft. The musculus biceps femoris is extraordinarily suitable for the transfer to the anterior part of the prosthesis part and thus facilitates the plastic covering. To cover the medial part of the prosthesis and to partly replace the function of a possibly resected musculus vastus medialis, the musculus sartorius is very suitable.

Muscle flap graft important for the stabilization and realignment of the patella

The muscle flap graft also plays a large role in the stabilization and realignment of the patella, especially when an extra-articular resection with replacement of the whole knee joint was necessary. For the plastic coverage of the prosthesis the execution of a primary gastrocnemius flap has been established as standard. Here, both the medial and the lateral portions are available, according to the resection.

PET attachment tube for secure refixation of the muscles and tendons to the prosthesis

To restore the active function of the knee joint secure fixation of the muscles and tendons to the prosthesis is particularly necessary after reconstruction of the proximal tibia. With the Mutars® system this works through the use of a PET attachment tube, which tightens around the prosthesis and is firmly sutured. This attachment tube is also conducive to the refixation of the gastrocnemius flap. Refixation of the ligamentum patellae combined with the gastrocnemius flap leads to very good functional results and to the restoration of active knee joint extension. A relevant weakness of the stretching apparatus, as often occurs after refixation of the ligaments directly to the prosthesis, can be prevented through use of the attachment tube.

Coverage of the muscle flap with use of a mesh graft, if tension-free skin closure impossible

Should a tension-free skin closure not be possible, especially in proximal tibia replacement, the additional coverage of the muscle flap with the use of “mesh graft” is unavoidable. Here, it is shown that the additional application of a vacuum bandage for 5 to 7 days can accelerate the growth of the transplanted skin.

The attachment tube is also applied in reconstruction of the capsule after proximal femur and proximal humerus resections (Fig. 5.7).

Capsule reconstruction and refixation of muscles and tendons with use of attachment tube

The attachment tube prevents the luxation of the prosthesis and has a stabilizing effect. Non-resected muscle groups and tendons can be sutured with the attachment tube and thus enables residual function of the corresponding joint. In this way, capsule reconstruction and refixation of muscles (especially the musculus gluteus medius) and tendons (tendon of the musculus iliopsoas) with the aid of the attachment tube are successful. The combination of a dual head prosthesis and an attachment tube leads to a maximization of the stability to be achieved and prevent postopera-

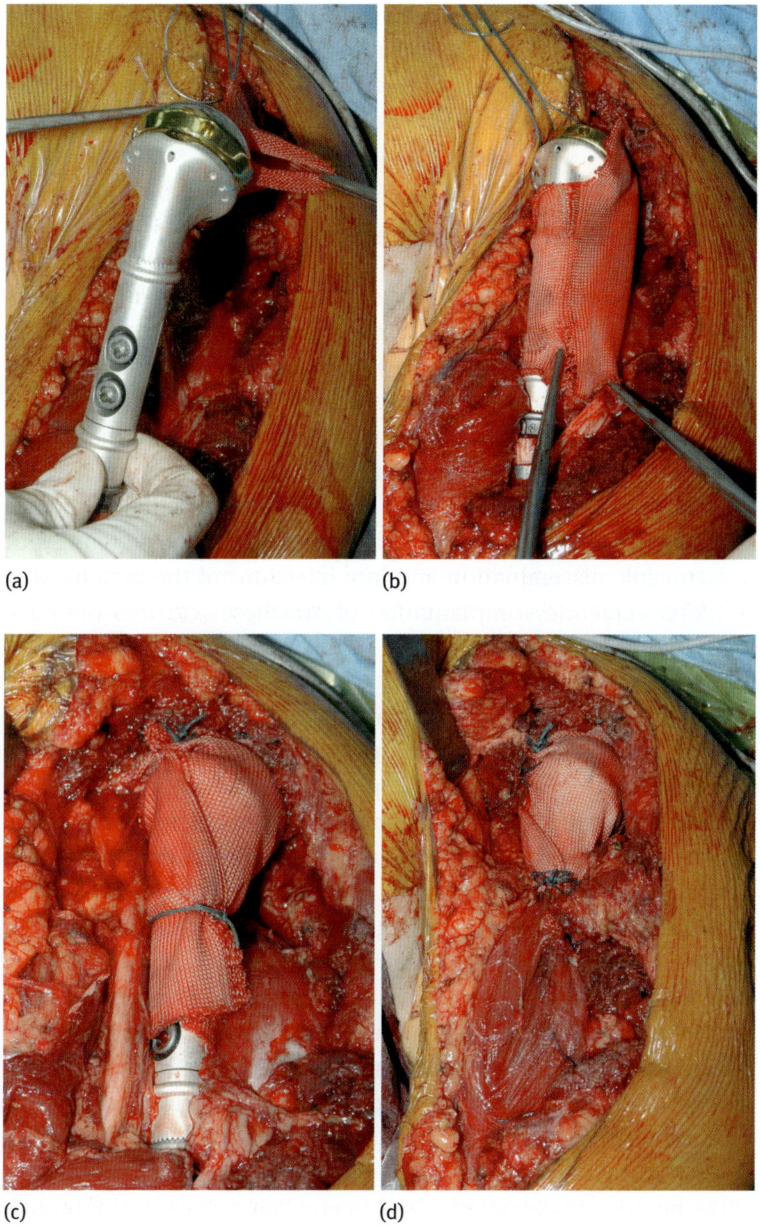

Fig. 5.7: Refixation of the muscles and tendons to the prosthesis by a PET attachment tube, which tightens around the prosthesis and is sutured firmly. (a) Silver-coated proximal humeral prosthesis that is fixed with Ethibond sutures (b) to the clavicula and scapular remains, (c) fixing the attachment tube to the prosthesis with Ethibond sutures and (d) covering the prosthesis with muscle, which is sutured to the attachment tube. The attachment tube serves the capsule reconstruction and the refixation of the remaining portions of the rotator cuffs, the musculus deltoideus and the long biceps tendon.

Prevention of postoperative luxations

tive luxations. In the replacement of the proximal humerus the attachment tube also serves capsule reconstruction and the refixation of the remaining parts of the rotator cuff of the musculus deltoideus and the long biceps tendon.

5.4 Postoperative Management

Peri- and postoperative prophylaxis with antibiotics

Peri- and postoperatively, all patients should be treated prophylactically with antibiotics (e.g., third-generation cephalosporins), at first intravenously for three days, then orally until completion of wound healing. However, on the basis of low numbers of cases of tumor endoprosthetics the published data are not verified here. In addition, all patients are informed that, as after a heart valve operation, in anticipated bacteremia (e.g., local infections or dental treatments) antibiotics prophylaxis should be conducted to prevent hematogenic dissemination and late infections of the prosthesis.

Immobilization, non-weight-bearing and/or weight-bearing and practice depending on the type and nature of the replacement

After cementless implantation of prostheses close to the knee joint, we recommend relatively strict immobilization and non-weight-bearing: six weeks partial weight-bearing of approximately 10 kg, followed by a slow increase in weight-bearing of approximately 5–10 kg per week (according to the patient's weight), until full weight-bearing is achieved. The practicing of mobility after distal femoral replacement should be limited, if a gastrocnemius flap was necessary to cover the defect (four weeks' immobilization with extension). In proximal tibia replacement immobilization with extension for approximately four weeks (e.g., in a Mecron splint) is essential, since the refixated gastrocnemius flap and the ligamentum patellae must first adhere to the attachment tube. From the fifth week postoperatively, the practice of flexion then begins. However, the maximal flexion should not exceed 90°, as otherwise a significantly premature wearing of the polyethylene groove has to be reckoned with.

In resections around the knee joint attention to and treatment of foot elevation weaknesses important

Currently, in resections that are close to the knee attention should be paid especially to a postoperatively occurring weakness of the muscles of the anterior and lateral compartments, i.e., elevation weakness of the feet. As the nervus peroneus is routinely visualized, it can result in slight damage by the hook pull or postoperative edema/hematoma. Slight pressure or pulling can lead to a disorder through the temporary disturbance of the microcirculation of the nerves. Just after reconstructions at the proximal tibia, there can also be limitation of foot elevation in cases of intact peroneus nerve through the resection and/or the replacement of the anterior musculature. If it should turn out to be a relative weakness and/or foot drop, efficient club foot prophylaxis with a peroneus feather is recommended. As a rule, functional disturbances are temporary and mostly restored within a few months.

Humeral reconstruction: exercising of elbow, wrist, and fingers to prevent contracture

Patients undergoing reconstruction of the proximal humerus are immobilized for 4–6 weeks in a Gilchrist bandage; however, exercising of the elbow and wrist as well as the finger is necessary prematurely, to prevent contractures.

Femur reconstruction: postoperative procedure dependent on use of a cemented or a non-cemented femoral stem

After reconstruction with a proximal femur replacement the postoperative procedure is dependent on whether a cemented or non-cemented femoral stem is chosen. In cemented femoral stems mobilization is mainly dependent on soft-tissue reconstruction. After initial postoperative bed rest for 2–3 days mobilization is often possible with pain-adapted full weight-bearing. In non-cemented femoral stems after initial bed rest for the first six weeks postoperatively, only partial weight-bearing is possible to initially guarantee osseointegration and hence sufficient stability of the stem. Here, the aforementioned recommendations for building up weight-bearing of prostheses around the knee joint are followed.

5.5 Function

Function result of tumor-/reconstruction prostheses characterized by loss of viable musculature
Assessment with the Enneking score (MSTS score)

The functional result of tumor prostheses and reconstruction prostheses is characterized to the highest extent by the loss of viable musculature. The result is measured in tumor orthopedics by the Enneking score, also called MSTS score. Here, both subjective parameters (pain, acceptance) and function parameters (range of movement, use of aids, gait displacement). A result of 100 % corresponds to an unlimited, free, and painless functioning of the affected extremity.

Best results with reconstructions of the proximal tibia (83 %) and the distal tibia (80 %)

We achieved the best results with reconstructions of the proximal tibia (83 %) (Fig. 5.8), followed by distal femur reconstruction, followed by distal femur reconstructions (80 %). Here, the patients can mostly flex the knee joint up to 90°, the active extension is often un limited, but can also be limited according to the extent of resection of the quadriceps musculature (Fig. 5.9).

Proximal femur replacement: approximately 70 % of normal function

Proximal humerus replacement: approximately 70 % of normal function

Patients with a proximal femur replacement aimed at an average of 70 % of normal function. Here, in older patients in particular, despite soft-tissue reconstruction of the gluteal musculature at the attachment tube, a Trendelenburg gait and in most cases the necessity for the use of an underarm crutch on the opposite site for longer walking distances was shown. In patients with reconstructions of the proximal humerus a value of 70 % is shown, mainly caused by the loss of function after resection of the nervus axillaris, whereby an abduction of 30° and an elevation over 60 %

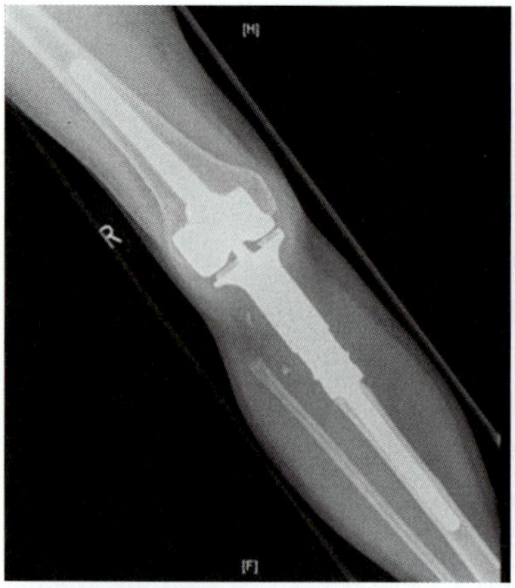

(a)

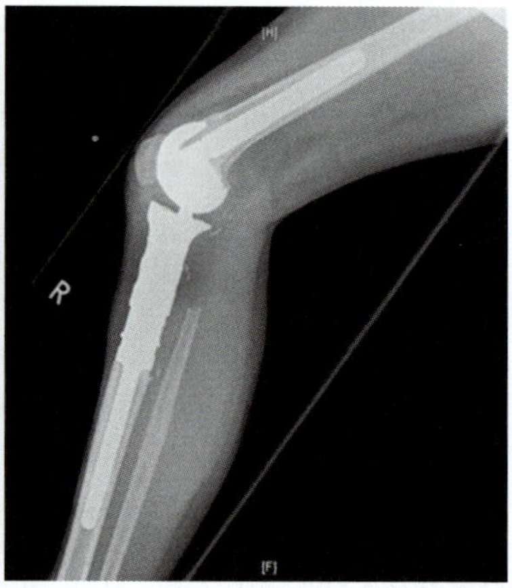

(b)

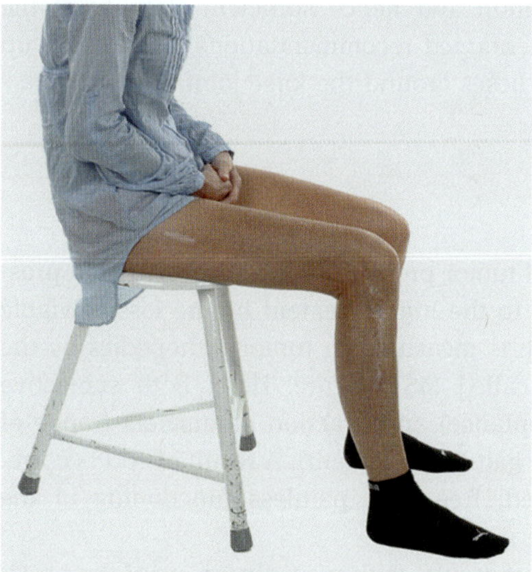

(c)

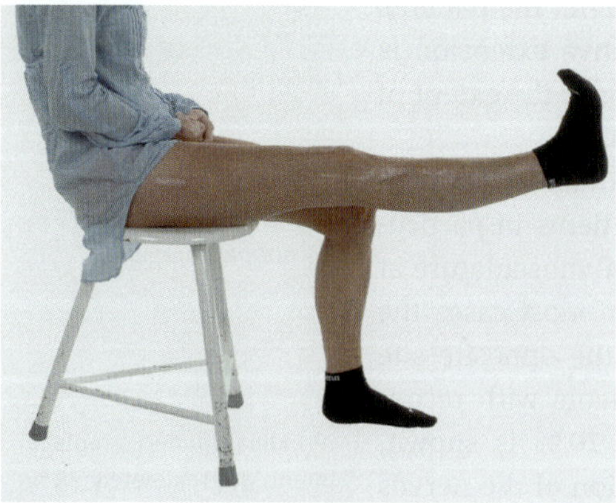

(d)

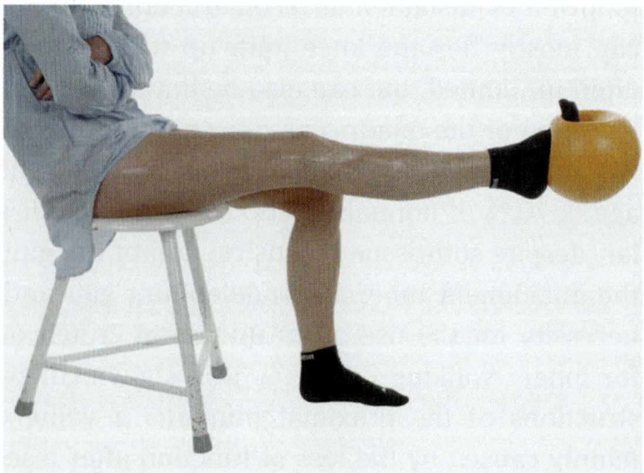

(e)

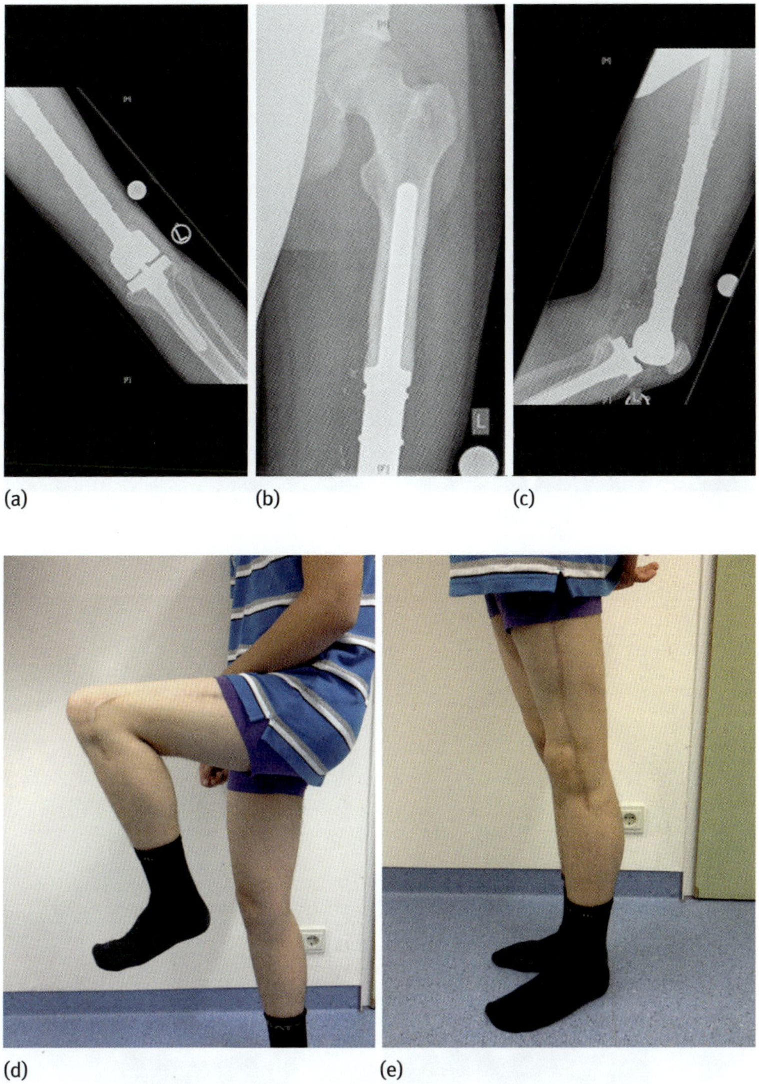

Fig. 5.9: Functional result after distal femur reconstructions (a–c). Here, the patients can mostly flex the knee joint up to 90° (d), the active extension is often unlimited (e).

◀ **Fig. 5.8:** Functional result with very good active extension ability (c–e) after implantation of a Mutars® prosthesis of the proximal tibia (a, b) and refixation of the extensor mechanism to the PET attachment tube.

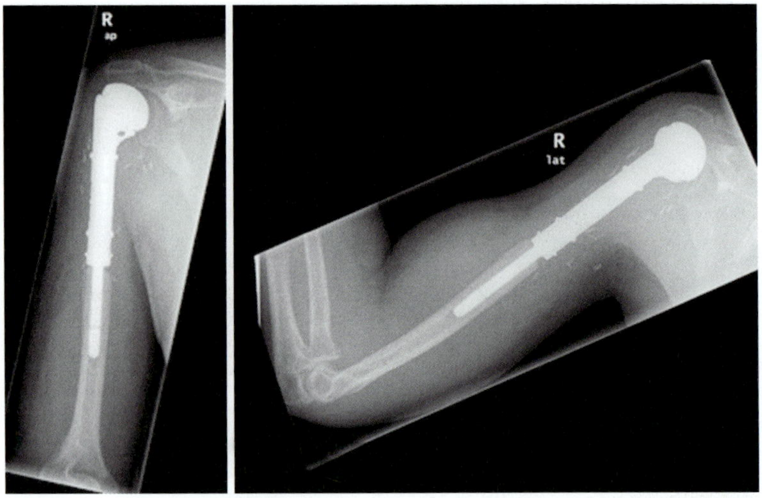

(a) (b)

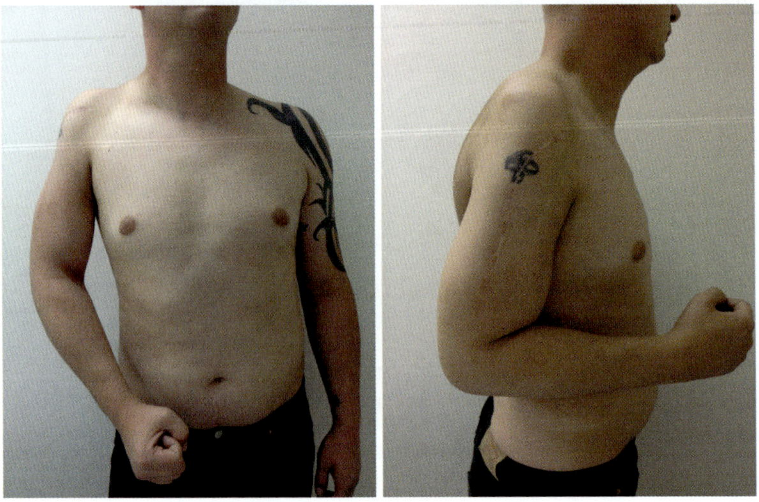

(c) (d)

Fig. 5.10: Functional result after reconstructions of the proximal humerus (a, b). Owing to the loss of function after resection of the nervus axillaris abduction over 30° (c) and an elevation over 60° (d) is difficult to achieve.

is difficult to achieve. Patients are however, in the situation to guide their hand to their mouth (Fig. 5.10).

Inverse proximal humerus prosthesis: active abduction up to approximately 90°

With use of an inverse tumor prosthesis of the proximal humerus, however, active abduction of at least 90° is expected (Fig. 5.11).

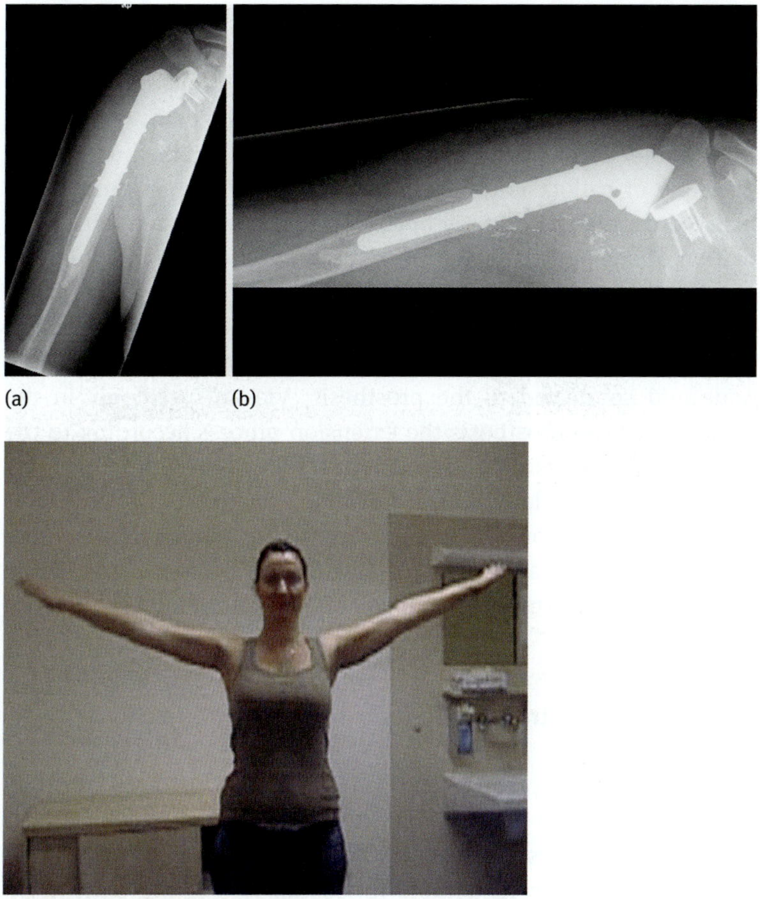

(a) (b) (c)

Fig. 5.11: In the case of preservation of the nervus axillaris and use of an inverse tumor prosthesis of the proximal humerus (a, b) active abduction up to 90° is mostly to be expected (c).

5.6 Special Prostheses

5.6.1 Growth Prostheses

A special indication for the tumor endoprosthetic provision is growth prostheses, which are applied in the reconstruction of bone defects in very young patients in whom a difference in leg length of more than 0.05 m is expected. Five to six years is the age limit for treatment with a growth prosthesis. As alternative treatment methods in even younger patients amputation and rotationplasty are referred to.

Growth prostheses in reconstructions of bone defects in very young patients

Alternatives: amputation and rotationplasty

Like tumor endoprostheses, modern growth prostheses are also modular and individually adaptable. In principle two forms of

Two forms of extendable prostheses
- With electromotor
- Principle of callotasis; with use of electromotor and extendable intramedullary nail

extendable prostheses are distinguished. On the one hand there are prostheses that are primarily equipped with an electromotor and lead to extension of the prosthesis due to induction. Here, the metallic prosthesis is extended; there is no bone gain.

Another form of the extendable prosthesis makes use of the principle of callotasis (Mutars® BioExpand). Here, a "dummy" is inserted during the primary operation that is expanded after completion of chemotherapy and the resulting difference in leg length of more than 0.03 m, in a second intervention using an electromotor and a extendable intramedullary nail in order to start the extension process. The extendable intramedullary nail is locked into the bone and connected to the prosthesis. Via an osteotomy in the stem area of the prosthesis the extension process according to the principle of callotasis with extension increments of 0.001 m per day up to the desired length. The advantage of this is that for later revision interventions in which very young patients have more bone matter available. The disadvantages comprise frequently appearing contractures, infections and implant failures.

5.6.2 Stump Construction Grafts

Stump construction graft:
- In hip exarticulation
- To preserve a functional stump for exoprosthesis

Because of tumor spread in the bones or soft tissue a hip exarticulation is sometimes unavoidable, where the lack of an amputation stump is the greatest problem in fitting an external prosthesis and consequently is a considerable functional loss to the patient. To preserve a functional stump and thereby give the patient the chance of having an exoprosthesis fitted, there is the possibility of stump construction grafts if there is sufficient soft-tissue coverage. Here, after resection of the whole femur an endoprosthetic proximal femur replacement with dual head is applied (Fig. 5.12). Because of the modularity of the Mutars® system the length of the stump can be varied and adapted to the soft-tissue situation. The remaining soft tissue can be fixed to the prosthesis with use of an attachment tube and enables a functional stump for adaptation of an exoprosthesis.

5.7 Complications

Most serious complication: local recurrence (rate: 1–9 %)

The most serious complication is local recurrence, which is accompanied by a very bad prognosis. The rate of local recurrence after extremity preservation with the use of tumor prostheses is given in the literature as 1 to 9 % and is comparable with ablative proce-

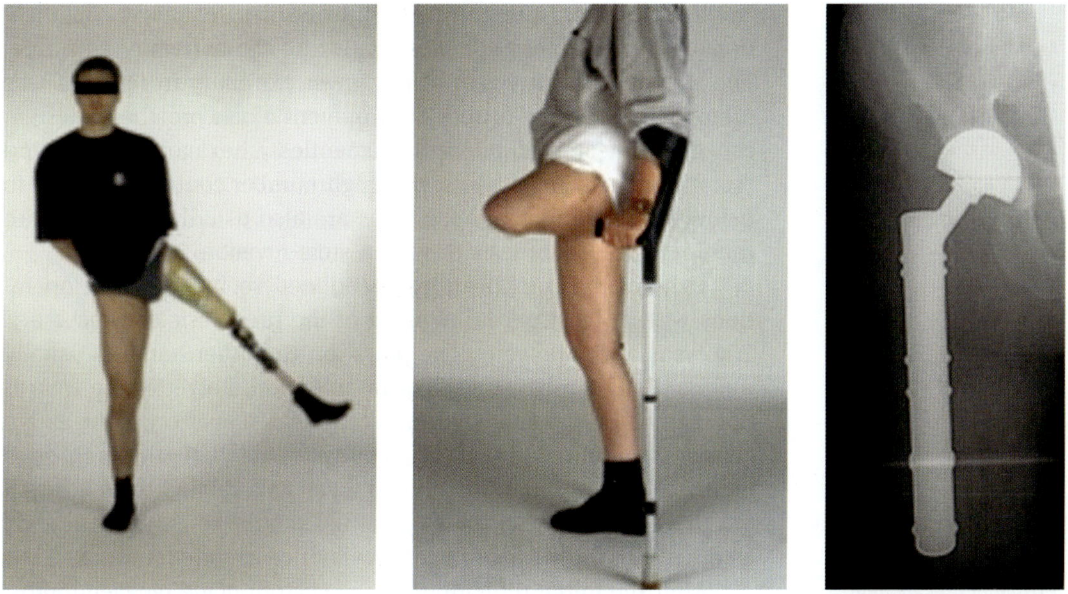

Fig. 5.12: After resection of the whole femur stump construction graft (a) with a Mutars® proximal femur prosthesis with dual head. With sufficient soft tissue coverage a functional stump (b) can be preserved through fixation of the musculature to the attachment tube over the prosthesis and thus a function stump can be formed to fit an exoprosthesis (c).

dures. However, to achieve such good results a wide resection is required, according to Enneking.

The 5- to 10-year survival rate of modern tumor prostheses lies between 69 and 90 %. The most frequent complications that make it necessary to explant the prosthesis are aseptic loosening, periprosthetic infection or periprosthetic fracture and/or stem fracture.

5- to 10-year survival rate of modern tumour prostheses 69–90 %

The infection rate at the lower extremity is up to 36 %, and is at its highest in reconstructions of the proximal tibia. In the case of a prosthesis infection, in primary endoprosthetics a two-stage revision with temporary implantation of an antibiotics-loaded bone cement spacer is unavoidable. In early infections (up to three weeks postoperatively) or the appearance of acute hematogenous infections (e.g., port infection) a one-stage procedure with debridement, lavage, and exchange of the polyethylene parts can be attempted. In up to 46 % of cases the periprosthetic infection of the tumor prosthesis leads to a secondary leg amputation. Increasingly over the last few years, the routine use of silver-coated prostheses (Mutars® Silver) has become established. The silver ions have the ability to lower infection rates, and so far do not seem to have any appreciable side effects. If an infection occurs despite silver coating, the secondary amputation rate up to now could be significantly reduced.

Infection:
- Rate approximately 36 % at the lower extremity
- Highest rate in proximal tibia reconstruction
- One- or two-stage revision
- Secondary amputation in approximately 46 %

Silver-coated prostheses lower infection rate

Aseptic loosening:
- Rate: approximately 8 %
- Treatable with preservation of the extremity

In contrast to periprosthetic infection, mechanical complications can be treated with preservation of the extremity as a rule. The aseptic loosening rate at the lower extremity in the past was up to 27 %. Owing to further development of the prosthesis design, especially the introduction of (cementless) hexagonal stems and "rotating hinge" knee joints, this high number could be reduced to below 8 %. Periprosthetic fractures are also usually treatable with the use of osteosynthesis or with a stem revision.

Periprosthetic fractures usually treatable

To treat the complications mentioned so far, complex operations with at least partial revision of the prosthesis are necessary. The wear of the polyethylene parts, on the other hand, is usually repairable by a relatively minor intervention. Polyethylene wear is not really a valid complication, but rather a side effect of the extensive use, particularly in young, active patients. It manifests through increasing instability of the joint as well as a related unsteady gait on uneven ground. An inlay exchange should be carried out early as otherwise the wear particles can induce aseptic loosening.

Polyethylene wear a side effect of extensive use

Inlay exchange as early as possible

Extremity preservation with modular prosthesis systems in bone tumors standard today

Rarely: amputations and rotationplasties

Indications, contraindications of the extremity preservation constantly changing

After the initial difficulties of the custom-made megaendoprostheses, these days, since the introduction of modular prosthesis systems, extremity preservation in bone tumors has become standard. Amputations and rotationplasties are only rarely necessary and the excellent functional results with modular prostheses lead to very high patient satisfaction. The continuous further developments in various materials, fixation systems, and coatings, as well as the growing experience of the surgeons, lead to a constantly expanding spectrum of applications of prostheses. Indications and contraindications for extremity preservation in tumor orthopedics are always changing, and should be reevaluated for each individual patient.

References

Campanacci M, Bacci G, Bertoni F, Picci P, Minutillo A, Franceschi C. The treatment of osteosarcoma of the extremities: twenty years' experience at the Istituto Ortopedico Rizzoli. Cancer 1981;48(7):1569–81. |

Dominkus M, Sabeti M, Toma C, Abdolvahab F, Trieb K, Kotz RI. Reconstructing the extensor apparatus with a new polyester ligament. Clin Orthop Relat Res 2006;453:32834.

Eckardt JJ, Eilber FR, Dorey FJ, Mirra JM. The UCLA experience in limb salvage surgery for malignant tumors. Orthopedics 1985;8(5):61221.

Favre, R, Pessereau, Delacroix, H, [2 Juvara Operations for Malignant Tumor of the Tibia and Femur.]. Bull Mem Soc Chir Paris, 1965. 55:15661.

Gosheger G, Goetze C, Hardes J, Joosten U, WinkelmannW, von Eiff C. The influence of the alloy of megaprostheses on infection rate. J Arthroplasty 2008;23(6):91620. Epub 13. 2. 2008.

Gosheger G, Gebert C, Ahrens H, Streitbuerger A, Winkelmann W, Hardes J. Endoprosthetic reconstruction in 250 patients with sarcoma. Clin Orthop Relat Res 2006;450:16471.

Gosheger G, Hardes J, Ahrens H, Streitburger A, Buerger H, Erren M, Gunsel A, Kemper FH, Winkelmann W, Von Eiff C. Silver-coated megaendoprostheses in a rabbit model an analysis of the infection rate and toxicological side effects. Biomaterials 2004;25(24):554756.

Gosheger G, Hillmann A, Lindner N, Rodl R, Hoffmann C, Burger H, Winkelmann W. Soft tissue reconstruction of megaprostheses using a trevira tube. Clin Orthop Relat Res 2001;393:26471.

Grimer RJ, Belthur M, Chandrasekar C, Carter SR, Tillman RM. Two-stage revision for infected endoprostheses used in tumor surgery. Clin Orthop Relat Res 2002:395:193203.

Grimer RJ, Carter SR, Tillman RM, Sneath RS, Walker PS, Unwin PS, Shewell PC. Endoprosthetic replacement of the proximal tibia. J Bone Joint Surg Br 1999;81(3):48894.

Ham SJ, Schraffordt Koops H, Veth RP, van Horn JR, Molenaar WM, Hoekstra HJ. Limb salvage surgery for primary bone sarcoma of the lower extremities: long-term consequences of endoprosthetic reconstructions. Ann Surg Oncol 1998;5(5):42336.

Hardes J, Ahrens H, Nottrott M, Dieckmann R, Gosheger G, Henrichs MP, Streitbürger A. Attachment tube for soft tissue reconstruction after implantation of a mega-endoprosthesis. Oper Orthop Traumatol 2012;24(3): 22734.

Hardes J, von Eiff C, Streitbuerger A, Balke M, Budny T, Henrichs MP, Hauschild G, Ahrens H. Reduction of periprosthetic infection with silvercoated megaprostheses in patients with bone sarcoma. J Surg Oncol 2010;101(5):38995.

Hardes J, Ahrens H, Gebert C, Streitbuerger A, Buerger H, Erren M, Gunsel A, Wedemeyer C, Saxler G, Winkelmann W, Gosheger G. Lack of toxicological sideeffects in silver-coated megaprostheses in humans. Biomaterials 2007;28(18):286975.

Hardes J, Gebert C, Schwappach A, Ahrens H, Streitburger A, Winkelmann W, Gosheger G. Characteristics and outcome of infections associated with tumor endoprostheses. Arch Orthop Trauma Surg 2006;126(5):28996.

Höll S, Schlomberg A, Gosheger G, Dieckmann R, Streitbuerger A, Schulz D, Hardes J. Distal femur and proximal tibia replacement with megaprosthesis in revision knee arthroplasty: a limb-saving procedure. Knee Surg Sports Traumatol Arthrosc 2012. Epub ahead of print 6. 3. 2012.

Jeys LM, Grimer RJ, Carter SR, Tillman RM. Risk of amputation following limb salvage surgery with endoprosthetic replacement, in a consecutive series of 1261 patients. Int Orthop 2003;27(3):1603.

Malawer MM, Chou LB. Prosthetic survival and clinical results with use of largesegment replacements in the treatment of high-grade bone sarcomas. J Bone Joint Surg Am 1995;77(8):115465.

Mittermayer F, Krepler P, Dominkus M, Schwameis E, Sluga M, Heinzl H, Kotz R. Long-term followup of uncemented tumor endoprostheses for the lower extremity. Clin Orthop Relat Res 2001;388:16777.

Shin DS, Weber KL, Chao EY, An KN, Sim FH. Reoperation for failed prosthetic replacement used for limb salvage. Clin Orthop Relat Res 1999;358:5363.

Tunn PU, Schmidt-Peter P, Pomraenke D, Hohenberger P. Osteosarcoma in children: long-term functional analysis. Clin Orthop Relat Res 2004; 421:2127.

Unwin PS, Cannon SR, Grimer RJ, Kemp HB, Sneath RS, Walker PS. Aseptic loosening in cemented custom-made prosthetic replacements for bone tumours of the lower limb. J Bone Joint Surg Br 1996;78(1):513.

R. Hube

6 Minimally Invasive Hip Endoprosthetics

6.1 General

With increasing acceptance of hip endoprosthetics, the indication for joint replacement in ever younger and more active patients is provided in order to preserve the accustomed quality of life despite irreversible damage to the hips. Thus, fast rehabilitation is also of increasing importance. Younger, professionally active patients can be reintegrated into social and professional life earlier through soft-tissue-conserving techniques.

Fast rehabilitation after hip joint replacement becoming more important

But also in older patients an accelerated mobilization is important, as immobilization with co-existing morbidities can lead to cardiovascular complications. This places enormous demands upon surgical technique, in order to achieve early functionality as far as possible with precise implantation of the components. Synonyms for these techniques are minimally invasive or mini-incision.

Elderly: immobilization with co-morbidities leads to cardiovascular complications

Reduced transgluteal approaches (so-called mini-incision) modified according to Bauer or Hardinge are lateral approaches and do not represent minimally invasive access as such, on the basis of access-induced injury of the gluteal musculature. Possible consequences are the at least temporary insufficiency of the gluteal musculature with typical Trendelenburg limp and the danger of damaging the nervus gluteus medius in necessary proximal extension. For this reason various authors have developed minimally invasive techniques to minimize soft tissue trauma. Among these are modified anterior, anterolateral, and posterolateral approaches (Fig. 6.1). Thus, reducing the size of the skin incision does not take priority, as defined by some authors, but the conservation of the musculature. The gluteal musculature is assigned special significance here, as it is the "motor of the hips" and essential for rehabilitation and the functioning of the hip joint. In this way, the early functionality is improved. Muscle insufficiencies should be reduced.

Mini-incision: reduced transgluteal approaches

Possible consequences:

- Temporary insufficiency of the gluteal musculature with Trendelenburg limp
- Injury to the nervus gluteus medius

Minimally invasive techniques to prevent soft-tissue trauma

Gluteal musculature "motor of the hips"

Through muscle-sparing preparation during the operation the blood loss and the connected transfusion rate are decreased compared with other conventional approaches. Further goals are to lower postoperative pain and if nothing else, shorten hospitalization without increasing complications.

Muscle-sparing preparation:

- Lower blood loss
- Lower pain
- Shorter hospitalization

Other proven approaches were modified and minimized. To this end, instruments were also adapted in order to facilitate

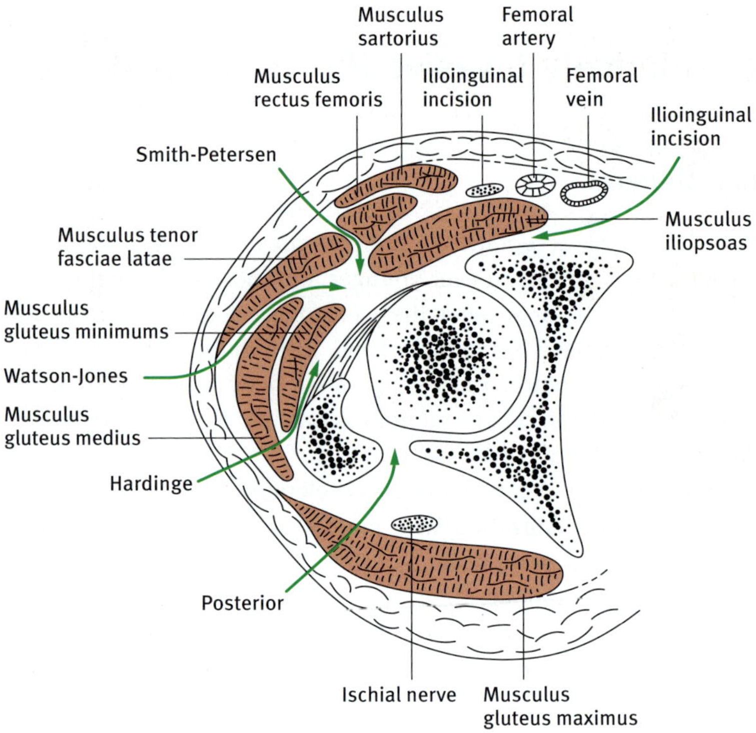

Fig. 6.1: Visualization of the individual approaches with their respective compartments. The transgluteal approaches according to Bauer and/or Hardinge do not conserve the gluteal musculature, while the other approaches choose anterior and posterior muscle compartments in order to damage the gluteal musculature as little as possible during the operation.

Minimized approach:
- Accelerated rehabilitation
- High-quality implantation
- Less soft-tissue trauma
- Lower frequency of luxation
- Increased cases of malpositioning

implantation via minimized approach in order to guarantee the reproducibility of the implantation and avoid complications. Currently, the accelerated rehabilitation possible requires high-quality implantation. The lower soft-tissue trauma compared with conventional approaches facilitates the revision situation in relation to the soft-tissue management. It is assumed that through this, risks such as luxation frequency can be reduced. However, it is important that the reproducibility of the implantation is not impaired. Thus, several cases of malpositioning of the components are described with minimally invasive techniques. This may lead not only to early complications, but also to impaired long-term results, for example, through increased wear in the case of steep positioning of the socket.

Modified instruments to simplify the implantation via minimized approach

To avoid this, modified instruments for rasping, reaming, and insertion were developed that enable simple insertion of the instruments like the definitive implants at the surgical site (Fig. 6.2). Here, too, care must be taken that the safety of the implantation is

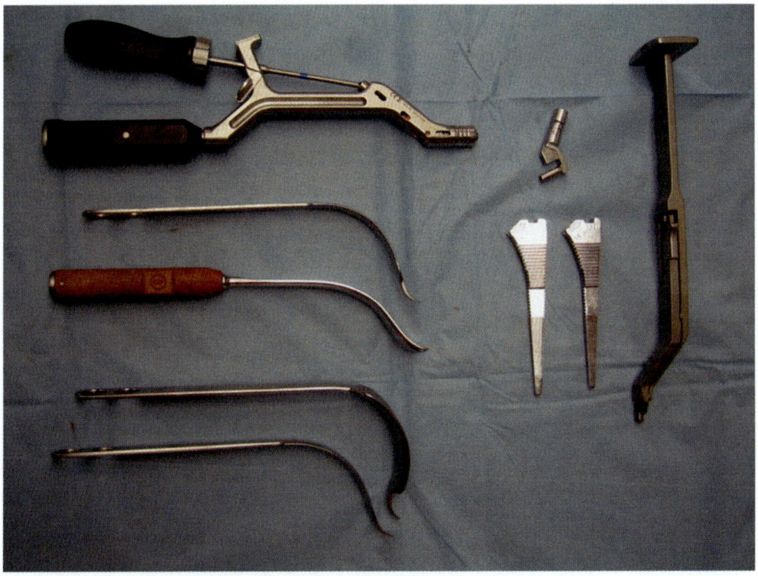

Fig. 6.2: Modified instruments and retractors for minimally invasive implantation techniques. The implantation is facilitated by the bent hand grips; impingement of the hand grips by the skin is prevented.

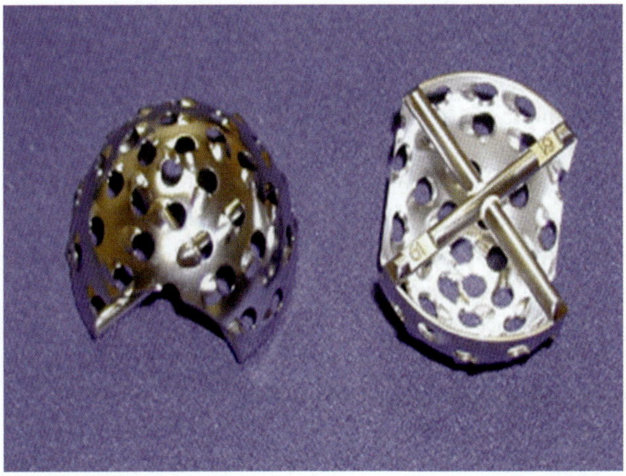

Fig. 6.3: Flattened actebular reamers for processing of the acetabulum in minimally invasive interventions. These can be inserted more easily at the surgical site because of the reduced volume. Owing to non-circumferential control they have a tendency toward conventional reaming rather than rejection at the preparation of the acetabulum.

not impaired. Thus, flattened acetabular reamers have a tendency toward eccentric processing of the socket bearing (Fig. 6.3). This can lead to impairment of the socket fixation and the resulting early failure.

Important: intensive physiotherapeutic exercise, adequate pain management

To be able to use the advantages of these approaches, intensive physiotherapeutic exercise and adequate pain management are necessary. Therefore, functional advantages, pain medication consumption, and patient satisfaction are required multifactorially, regardless of the length of the skin incision. In this way minimally invasive hip endoprosthetics is not only to be understood as a change in surgical technique, but also as an interdisciplinary process.

6.2 Patient Selection

Aims of minimally invasive approaches:
- Reduction of surgical trauma
- Broad spectrum of indications
- No contraindications

The aim of minimally invasive approach is to reduce surgical trauma without limiting the exposure of the femur and acetabulum to guarantee a reproducible implantation. But the aim should also be a broad spectrum of indications and the absence of any possible contraindications. This means that the approach must be able to adapt to the anatomy of the individual patients and the resulting surgical requirements. Above all, the extension in problem situations is essential. Furthermore, the approach should permit the use of all the usual implants, including cemented fixation.

Strict patient selection on the learning curve

Exclusion of obese or very muscular patients

Currently on the learning curve, patients should be strictly selected for minimally invasive operations. Obese or very muscular patients should be excluded. This also applies to preoperative hip joints or malalignment of the proximal femur or in the area of the acetabulum, such as for example severe dysplasia or ankylotic situations. With increasing experience at each technique used, the indication can be expanded. Principally, there are no main contraindications with sufficient experience, since anterolateral and posterolateral approaches are currently easily extendable.

6.3 The Posterolateral Approach

Posterolateral approach:
- Most frequently used approach worldwide
- Muscle-sparing
- Increased luxation rate

The posterior approach in the recovery position of the patient is the approach most used worldwide. It is very muscle-sparing per se, as it bypasses the gluteal musculature posteriorly (Fig. 6.4). But the musculus piriformis must be detached in most cases and is refixed after implantation of the hip endoprosthesis (Fig. 6.5). In addition, the trauma of the short external rotators can be reduced through minimization of the access. The problem of the posterolateral approach with regard to an increased luxation rate is a significant disadvantage. Through better refixation techniques of the posterior capsule and the short external rotators the luxation rate could be significantly improved. However, it continues to be shown

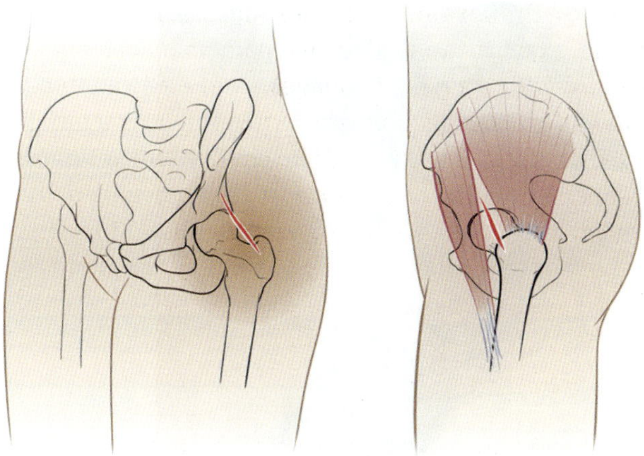

Fig. 6.4: Visualization of the posterolateral approaches at the muscle level. Even in conventional incision control the approach spares the gluteal musculature, since it is bypassed dorsally. A further reduction in the incision control under continuing sparing of the short external rotators and partly even the musculus piriformis can further reduce the muscle trauma.

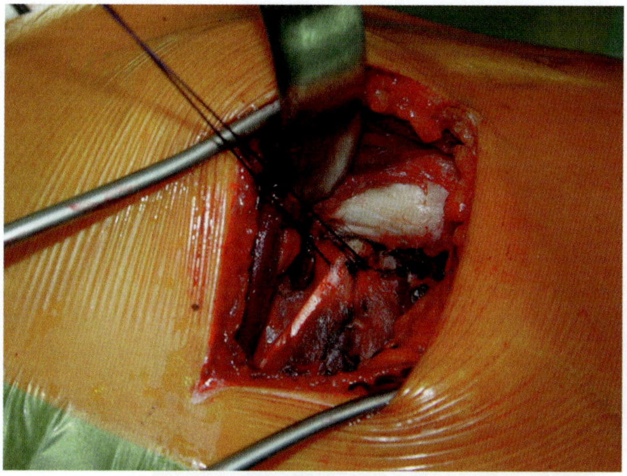

Fig. 6.5: lateral approach. After implantation of the hip endoprosthesis the muscle attachment is refixed.

to be raised compared with anterior and anterolateral approaches. Here, anterior and anterolateral approaches provide a useful initiative.

▸ Gradual reduction of the approach

One of the greatest advantages of the posterior approach is the possibility of gradually reducing the access. This can significantly minimize the learning curve. Also, with smaller access both the socket and the proximal femur are very well visualized (Figs. 6.6 and 6.7). For some authors, however, only the skin incision is

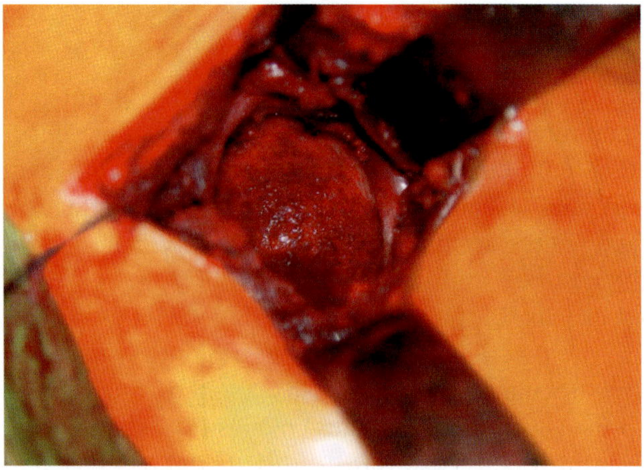

Fig. 6.6: Visualization of the acetabulum via a posterolateral anterior approach. The number of retractors is limited to a minimum, since they themselves require space: the insertion of more retractors would reduce the working space further.

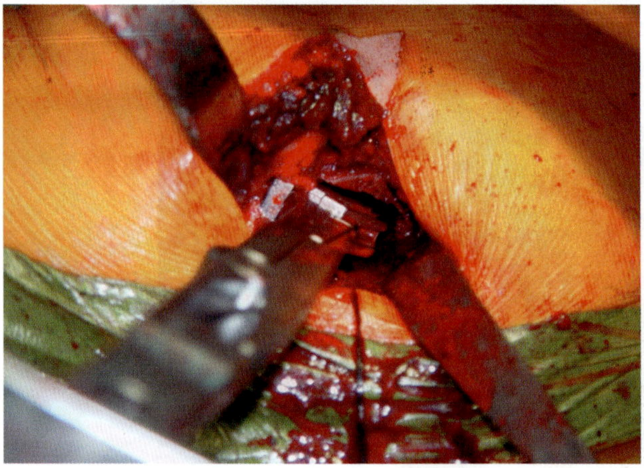

Fig. 6.7: Visualization of the proximal femur with rasp found in situ for a straight stem. With use of the posterolateral approach the implantation of a straight stem is a problem-free surgical technique.

After 6–12 weeks hardly any difference between conventional and minimally invasive approach

changed. Dorr et al. show on the other hand fewer pain symptoms, better function, as well as shorter inpatient treatment postoperatively. For all studies it is the same that after 6–12 weeks the clinical results between conventional and minimally invasive approaches are similar.

6.4 The Anterolateral Approach

The anterolateral approach is defined by the Watson-Jones interval between the musculus gluteus medius and the musculus tensor fasciae latae (Fig. 6.8). Currently in central Europe, this, the most frequently used muscle-sparing approach, had the advantage of good presentation of the acetabulum and femur and can be carried out in both the posterior and lateral positions (OCM approach). A slightly arched incision of the fascia significantly facilitates detection of the interval. After digital preparation of the intermuscular septum the intra-articular capsule is visualized. As the anterior portion of the capsule is contracting because of existing external rotation–flexion–contracture in coxarthrosis, this should be excised at the access. It is a part of pathology. It is important that the excision is limited to only the anterior portion of the capsule, in order to preserve soft-tissue tension. To determine the femoral neck osteotomy the trochanter minor normally serves as a reference. This is not palpable from anterolateral and anterior approaches without expansion; thus, the fossa trochanterica is used as the exit point of the osteotomy. According to the anatomy and in accordance with preoperative planning with the stem used, the gradient of the osteotomy is determined by this exit point.

Anterolateral approach:
- In the Watson-Jones interval
- Most frequent approach in Europe
- Muscle-sparing
- Good presentation of acetabulum and femur
- In the posterior and lateral position

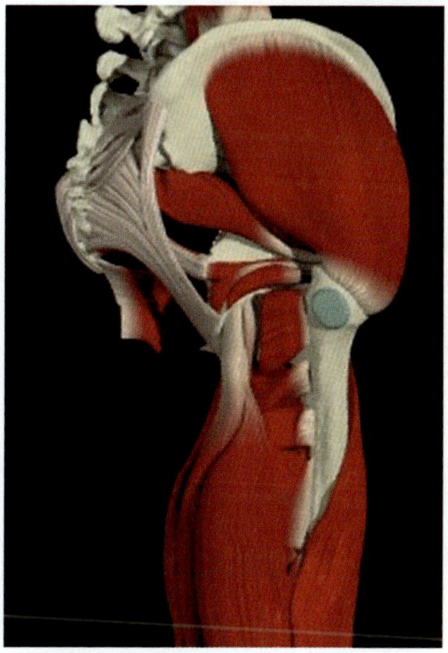

Fig. 6.8: Visualization of the muscle interval in the anterolateral approach between the musculus gluteus medius and the musculus tensor fasciae latae. With the correct surgical method the musculature is relaxed during the operation owing to special positioning techniques. Muscle damage during the visualization of acetabulum and proximal femur is minimized.

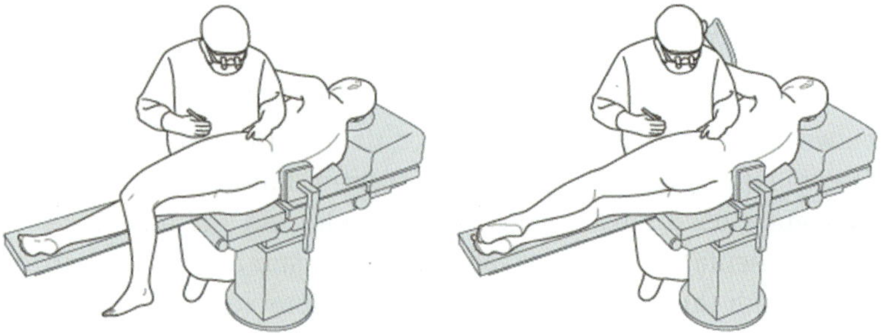

Fig. 6.9: Position of the patient and surgeon while the anterolateral approach is carried out in the lateral position. For the stem implantation (left) the leg is positioned in hyperextension, swinging out, and adduction. For the skin incision and socket preparation (right) both legs are positioned on top of each other.

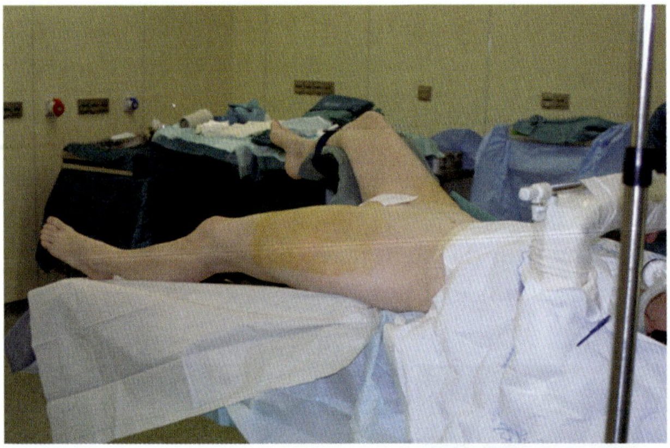

Fig. 6.10: Positioning of a patient to carry out anterolateral approach in supine position. The leg to be operated on is swung back with the aid of the operation table, so that a hyperextension is possible in order to visualize the proximal femur. The contralateral leg is positioned outward so that there is no disturbance during the stem implantation from the necessary swinging out and adduction of the operated leg. This positioning can also be carried out for the anterior approach, if no extension table is used.

Exposition of the proximal femur through hyperextension

Expansion of the approach in complications and revision surgery without confusion of vascular and nerve structures possible

A problem of anterior and anterolateral approaches is the exposure of the proximal femur. This is achieved through hyperextension of the femur. Through this, the gluteal musculature is transposed dorsally and the 20ztexposure of the proximal femur enabled. In the lateral position this is easier with better hyperextension of the leg to be operated upon. The leg is maintained in 90° external rotation, adduction, and hyperextension during visualization (Fig. 6.9). Thus, no tendon notch should occur in muscular patients. The lateral position is disadvantageous for the untrained, which somewhat impedes the exact position of the socket components, as does examination of the correct leg length.

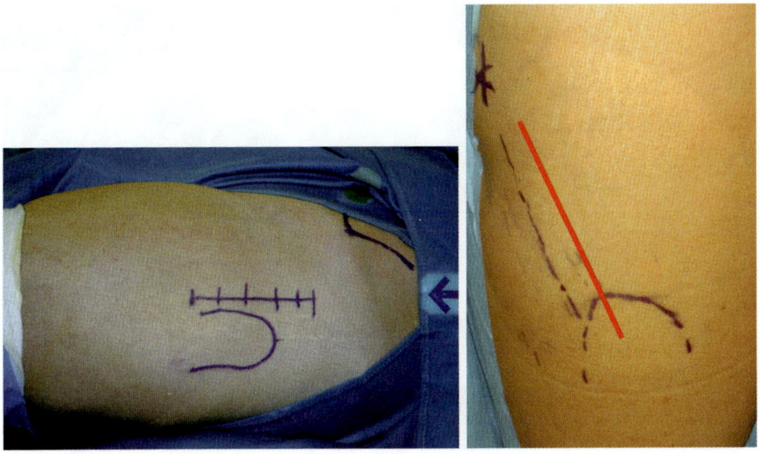

(a) (b)

Fig. 6.11: Visualization of the skin incisions for anterolateral approaches in supine (a) and lateral (b) positions. Because of the various possibilities of both positions to hyperextend the operated leg, the skin incision is also chosen differently by most surgeons. With the lateral approach it is rather skewed. This corresponds to the lengthening of the stem axis at exploration of the proximal femur.

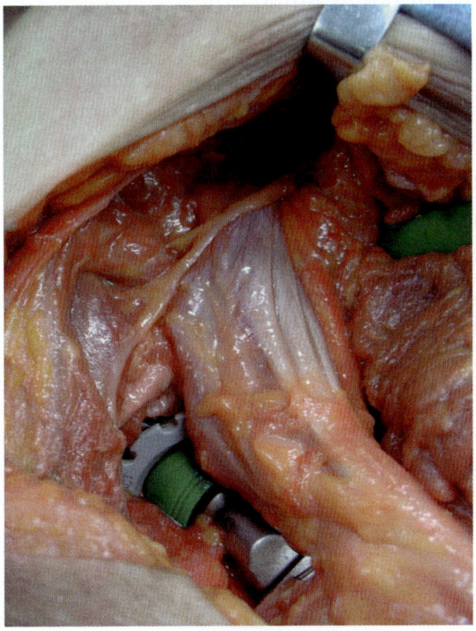

Fig. 6.12: Intraoperative site of the hip joint after implantation of test prostheses. The motor ramus of the nervus gluteus superior for the musculus tensor fasciae latae crosses at the proximal end of the muscle interval.

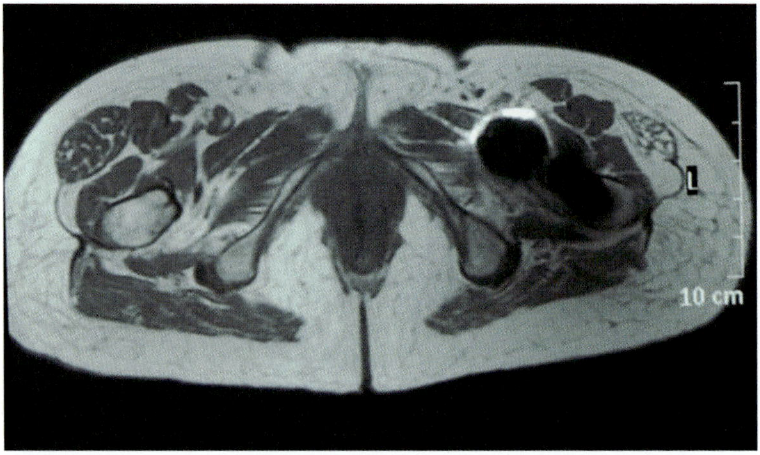

Fig. 6.13: MRT of both hip joints, left after implantation of a hip joint total endoprosthesis via an anterolateral approach: the fatty degeneration of the musculus tensor fasciae latae through damage of the motor tensor ramus of the nervus gluteus superior is shown clearly on the left.

In a supine position hyperextension is achieved by swinging the leg out (Fig. 6.10). Because of the different leg positions in the supine and/or lateral position for the visualization of the femur, the skin incision is also carried out in different ways by most surgeons (Fig. 6.11). Visualization of the socket is comparable in both positions.

Watson-Jones interval is not an interneural interval

An advantage is that the approach in complications management and in revision surgery without confusion of vascular and nerve structures can be expanded proximally and distally. It is disadvantageous that with the Watson-Jones interval it is not an interneural interval, as both muscles are innervated by the nervus gluteus superior. The motor ramus for the tensor fasciae latae crosses at the proximal end of the muscle interval, approximately 0.04 m above the trochanter major (Fig. 6.12). In non-preoperated hips this can be digitally displaced proximally and repeatedly spared. If the nerve has sustained damage, fatty degeneration of the musculus tensor fasciae latae occurs (Fig. 6.13).

6.5 The Anterior Approach

Anterior approach:
- In the Smith-Petersen interval

The anterior approach is carried out in the Smith-Peterson interval, between the musculus sartorius and the musculus tensor fasciae latae. The operation takes place in supine position either with slight swinging out of the leg or with the aid of the extension table for better display of the proximal femur. The exploration of the socket is good; that of the proximal femur in muscular patients is problematic, mainly when straight stems are applied. Just the pressure of the hook on the musculus tensor fasciae latae can, as described by various authors, lead to significant injury of the muscle.

- Socket exploration good, femur exploration problematic

Compared with the anterolateral approach, it is an advantage that it also concerns an interneural interval. The anterior muscle groups are supplied by the nervus femoralis, the laterally situated ones by the nervus gluteus superior. Thus, in the deep layers no nerve damage is expected. The frequent injury of the nervus cutaneous femoris lateralis with the use of the anterior approach, which in various anatomical variations runs partly laterally, is problematic. Via a modified, more laterally located skin incision the risk of a nerve lesion can be reduced.

- Approach through the interneural interval
- Frequent damage of the nervus cutaneous femoris lateralis

Expansion distally and proximally without further damage of the nervus cutaneous femoris lateral is problematic. Here, the postero- and anterolateral approaches are advantageous. Also, the visualization of the proximal femur is more difficult than with other approaches; thus, these limitations significantly limit the approach in complications management and in revision surgery. The higher complication rate described could be lowered through improvement in technique, the instruments, and the implant choice used.

- Expansion distally and proximally problematic
- Limited approach in complications and revision surgery

6.6 Effect of the Approach on the Choice of Implant

When considering the numbers of implantations of hip stems, it is noticeable that, despite very good results with straight stems, shorter implants are increasingly used. With these implants the trochanter major has to be visualized in only a limited way. The soft-tissue-sparing implantation because of the varus preparation medial to the fossa trochanterica with just minimally invasive techniques is significantly simplified (Figs. 6.14, 6.15). This is certainly a reason for these implants being increasingly chosen. Thus, the adapted soft-tissue techniques have certainly profoundly changed the choice of implants over the past few years.

Increasing use of shorter implants in minimally invasive techniques

6.7 Marketing or Benefit?

Hip endoprosthesis is one of the most successful surgical methods in the whole field of surgery. These results to which all innovations must be oriented were achieved with standard approaches. The aims of these approaches are good visualization of the surgical

Hip endoprosthetics one of the most successful surgical methods

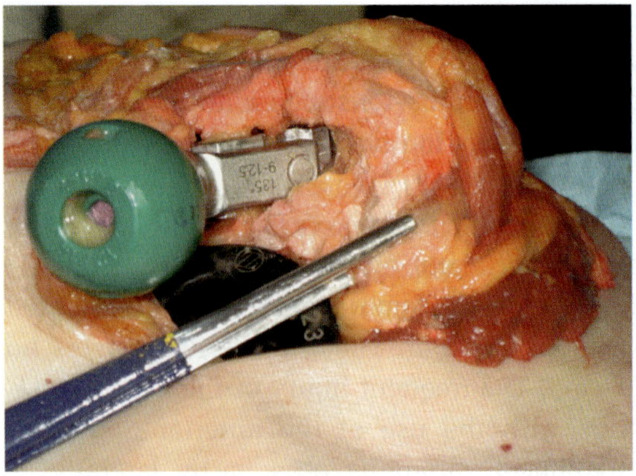

Fig. 6.14: Surgical site with visualization of the proximal femur after implantation of the test stem for a so-called short stem: the greater trochanter is not discriminated by the stem. The preparation takes place medial to the fossa trochanterica. Visualization is significantly simplified in minimally invasive surgical techniques.

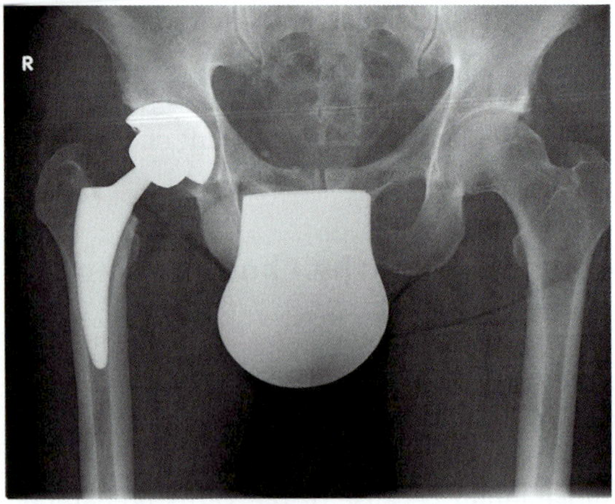

Fig. 6.15: Pelvic X-ray of the condition after right-sided implantation of a modern stem system after minimally invasive implantation. The greater trochanter is not damaged by the preparation.

field, expandability, the absence of specific complications and of course soft-tissue sparing too.

Less aseptic loosening

Increasing functional problems: impingement, luxation, leg length differences

With the introduction of modern tribological pairings the problem of aseptic loosening because of particle sickness can be significantly reduced. Increasingly function problems are coming to the foreground, such as impingement, luxations, and leg length differences. In the search for approaches, minimally invasive techniques with soft-tissue sparing represent an approach to reducing luxation. On the other hand, through the reduction in visualization

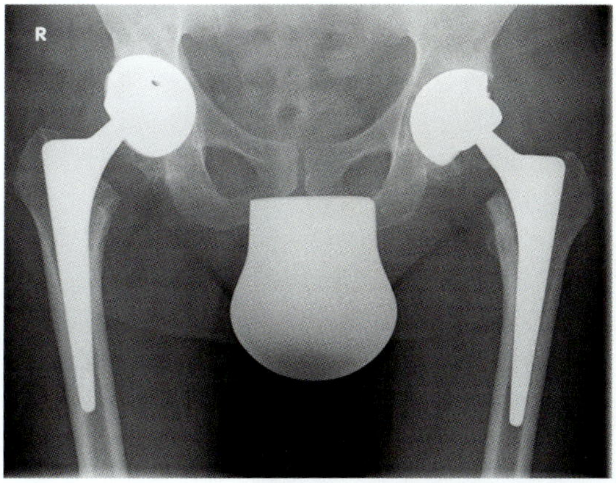

Fig. 6.16: Pelvic X-ray of the condition after bilateral implantation. The steep position of both sockets is clearly shown. The straight stem on the right is a varus implantation.

there is a danger of malpositioning of the implant (Fig. 6.16). There is a danger of an increase in the complication rate.

Minimally invasive techniques:
- Soft-tissue sparing
- Less luxation
- More malpositioning
- Higher complication rate
- Apart from smaller skin incision and lower blood loss, no advantages compared with conventional approaches
- Significantly more damage to the nervus cutaneous femoris lateralis

Despite partially insufficient study and the lack of evidence of the proposed advantages, these techniques have become widespread within a very short time. Almost all clinics advertise on their website with appropriate data. Thus, in the meta-analysis by Smith et al. with evaluation of 28 studies, apart from the reduced skin incision and lower blood loss, no advantages compared with conventional approaches were shown. In the same work a significantly higher incidence of injuries to the nervus cutaneous femoris lateralis was the resulting complication. In spite of these data these techniques and the proposed advantages are still promoted, although there is mostly no evidence for these. In the long term, however, these techniques will only become established if a lasting improvement in the quality of provision is achieved.

6.8 Summary

Useful reduction of the trauma in the implantation of hip endoprostheses

The decrease in the trauma of implantation of hip endoprostheses is useful, especially of the abductors as the engine of the hips. Here, it is vital that proven principles are not abandoned. Just the preoperative planning is assigned an even greater significance in a limited approach. Intraoperatively, the structures to be addressed, such as the muscle interval, osteotomy planes, etc., can be identified with certainty.

The expected use of the minimally invasive hip endoprosthetics, however, owing to the reduced approach, is nevertheless

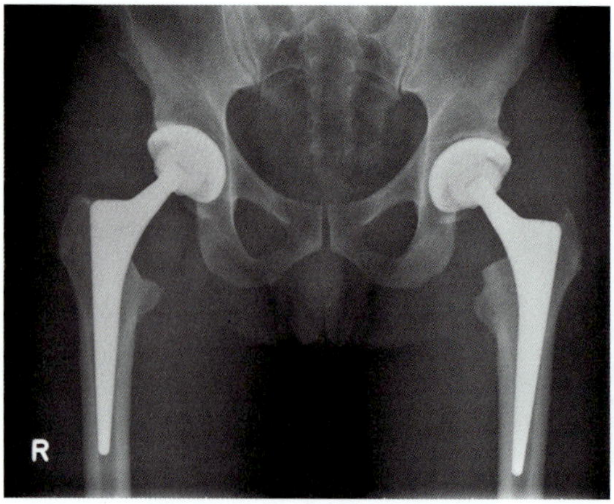

Fig. 6.17: Pelvic X-ray of the condition after bilateral implantation of cementless hip joint total endoprostheses after minimally invasive implantation. The false osteotomy plane on both sides appears because of an inadequate intraoperative visualization.

Benefit of a minimally invasive approach proven

Risk with smaller approaches and adjustment of the approach also documented

In the middle and long term no advantage compared with conventional approaches

accompanied by potential risks. Proposed benefits such as reduced muscle trauma, smaller scars, lower blood loss and pain, shorter hospitalization and rehabilitation, and improved satisfaction rate were proven in various studies. But the risks due to smaller approaches and above all the adjustment of paths of approach, such as increased complications, worse component positioning, and trauma of the unindicated structures are documented (Fig. 6.17). Muscular patients are difficult to operate upon. It is also to be expected that the functional results converge with those of conventional approaches in the middle and long term. Further examinations are pending.

Minimization of complications through defensive spectrum of indications and adequate skin incision

The possible complications described, with the significant learning curve, the stress on unindicated soft tissue, and malpositioning, however, are minimized through a defensive spectrum of indications and adequate skin incision in accordance with the surgeon's own experience of these specific surgical techniques. Thus, the resulting clinical problems such as luxation, impingement, leg length differences or offset problems can largely be avoided even in the learning curve. Sufficient exploration and expandability are vital for the quality of an approach. Whichever approach is chosen by the surgeon at the time, it should be as minimally invasively operated as possible, but as invasive as necessary to be reproducible. This lies with the responsibility of the individual. Only in this way are the known long-term results guaranteed, with very good satisfaction rates in hip endoprosthetics, and possibly further improved. To address the complications and in the revision field,

Approach as minimally invasive as possible, but as invasive as necessary

Table 6.1: Illustration of the suitability of individual minimally invasive techniques with regard to implantation, expansion, revision capability, and soft-tissue sparing.

	anterior	a/l R	a/l S	Bauer	posterior
Stem implantation	+	++	+++	+++	+++
Socket implantation	++	+++	+++	+++	++
Expansion		++	++	+++	+++
Revision	+	++	+++	+++	+++
Soft tissue	++	++	++		++
Total	+	++	+++	++	+++

various approaches should be mastered by the surgeon, especially in view of the treatment of periprosthetic infections. An evaluation of approaches with regard to visualization, expandability, revision capability, and soft-tissue sparing is shown in Table 6.1.

References

Bal BS, Haltom D, Aleto T, Barrett M. Early complications of primary total hip replacement performed with a two-incision minimally invasive technique. Surgical technique. J Bone Joint Surg Am 2006;88(Suppl 1 Pt 2): 221–33.

Bennett D, Ogonda L, Elliott D, Humphreys L, Lawlor M, Beverland D. Comparison of immediate postoperative walking ability in patients receiving minimally invasive and standard-incision hip arthroplasty: a prospective blinded study. J Arthroplasty 2007;22(4):490–5.

Berger RA, Jacobs JJ,Meneghini RM, Della Valle C, Paprosky W, Rosenberg AG. Rapid rehabilitation and recovery with minimally invasive total hip arthroplasty. Clin Orthop Relat Res 2004;429:239–47.

Bertin KC, Röttinger H. Anterolateral mini-incision hip replacement surgery: a modified Watson-Jones approach. Clin Orthop Relat Res 2004;429: 248–55.

Dixon MC, Scott RD, Schai PA, Stamos V. A simple capsulorrhaphy in a posterior approach for total hip arthroplasty. J Arthroplasty 2004;19(3): 373–6.

Dorr LD, Maheshwari AV, Long WT, Wan Z, Sirianni LE. Early pain relief and function after posterior minimally invasive and conventional total hip arthroplasty. A prospective, randomized, blinded study. J Bone Joint Surg Am 2007;89(6):1153–60.

Dorr LD, Thomas D, Long WT, Polatin PB, Sirianni LE. Psychologic reasons for patients preferring minimally invasive total hip arthroplasty. Clin Orthop Relat Res 2007;458:94–100.

Goosen JH, Kollen BJ, Castelein RM, Kuipers BM, Verheyen CC. Minimally invasive versus classic procedures in total hip arthroplasty: a double-blind randomized controlled trial. Clin Orthop Relat Res 2011;469(1): 200–8.

Graw BP, Woolson ST, Huddleston HG, Goodman SB, Huddleston JI. Minimal incision surgery as a risk factor for early failure of total hip arthroplasty. Clin Orthop Relat Res 2010;468(9):2372–6.

Hartzband MA. Posterolateral minimal incision for total hip replacement: technique and early results. Orthop Clin North Am 2004;35(2):119–29.

Howell JR, Masri BA, Duncan CP. Minimally invasive versus standard incision anterolateral hip replacement: a comparative study. Orthop Clin North Am 2004;35(2):153–62.

Kennon R, Keggi J, Zatorski LE, Keggi KJ. Anterior approach for total hip arthroplasty: beyond the minimally invasive technique. J Bone Joint Surg Am 2004;86(A Suppl 2):91–7.

Laffosse JM, Chiron P, Molinier F, Bensafi H, Puget J. Prospective and comparative study of the anterolateral mini-invasive approach versus minimally invasive posterior approach for primary total hip replacement. Early results. Int Orthop 2007;31(5):597–603.

Matta JM, Ferguson TA. The anterior approach for hip replacement. Orthopedics 2005;28(9):927–8.

McGrory BJ, Finch ME, Furlong PJ, Ruterbories J. Inzision length correlates with patient weight, height, and gender when using a minimal-incision technique in total hip arthroplasty. J Surg Orthop Adv 2008;17(2):77–81.

Meneghini RM, Pagnano MW, Trousdale RT, Hozack WJ. Muscle damage during MIS total hip arthroplasty: Smith-Petersen versus posterior approach. Clin Orthop Relat Res 2006;453:293–8.

Ogonda L, Wilson R, Archbold P, Lawlor M, Humphreys P, O'Brien S, Beverland D. A minimal-incision technique in total hip arthroplasty does not improve early postoperative outcomes. A prospective, randomized, controlled trial. J Bone Joint Surg Am 2005;87(4):701–10.

Parratte S, Pagnano MW. Muscle damage during minimally invasive total hip arthroplasty: cadaver-based evidence that it is significant. Instr Course Lect 2008;57:231–4.

Parvizi J, Sharkey PF, Pour AE, Rapuri V, Hozack WJ, Rothman RH. Hip arthroplasty with minimally invasive surgery: a survey comparing the opinion of highly qualified experts vs patients. Arthroplasty 2006;21 (6 Suppl 2):38–46.

Picado CH, Garcia FL, Marques W Jr. Damage to the superior gluteal nerve after direct lateral approach to the hip. Clin Orthop Relat Res 2007;455:209–11.

Pospischill M, Kranzl A, Attwenger B, Knahr K. Minimally invasive compared with traditional transgluteal approach for total hip arthroplasty: a comparative gait analysis. J Bone Joint Surg Am 2010;92(2):328–37.

Röttinger H. The MIS anterolateral approach for THA.Orthopäde 2006; 35(7):708, 710–5.

Siguier T, Siguier M, Brumpt B. Mini-incision anterior approach does not increase dislocation rate: a study of 1037 total hip replacements. Clin Orthop Relat Res 2004;426:164–73.

Smith TO, Blake V, Hing CB. Minimally invasive versus conventional exposure for total hip arthroplasty: a systematic review and meta-analysis of clinical and radiological outcomes. Int Orthop 2011;35(2):173–84.

Svensson O, Sköld S, Blomgren G. Integrity of the gluteus medius after the transgluteal approach in total hip arthroplasty. J Arthroplasty 1990;5(1): 57–60.

Von Roth P, Olivier M, Preininger B, Perka C, Hube R. BMI and gender do not influence surgical accuracy during minimally invasive total hip arthroplasty. Hip Int 2011;21(6):688–93.

Wan Z, Boutary M, Dorr LD. The influence of acetabular component position on wear in total hip arthroplasty. J Arthroplasty 2008;23(1):51–6.

Wohlrab D, Droege JW, Mendel T, Brehme K, Riedl K, Leuchte S, Hein W. Minimally invasive vs. transgluteal total hip replacement. A 3-month follow-up of a prospective randomized clinical study. Orthopade 2008;37(11): 1121–6.

Woo RY, Morrey BF. Dislocations after total hip arthroplasty. J Bone Joint Surg Am 1982;64(9):1295–306.

H. Kiefer

7 Navigation in Endoprosthetics

7.1 Introduction

Computer-assisted operations have been used in joint endoprosthetics since the mid-1990s with the aim of improving the precision of the implantation and thus the treatment results for the patient. Therefore, the notion of precision, in principle monitors the revised positioning and choice of joint endoprosthetic components by the surgeon.

Computer-assisted operations to improve treatment results

The simplest form of computer assistance are today established procedures for preoperative planning. The most elaborate form was the use of surgical robots at the end of the 1990s, which on the basis of a CT dataset, reamed a preoperatively fixed implant position for cementless hip stems and later also knee endoprostheses in the bone. The advantage of better and preoperatively precisely planned implant positioning was countered by the disadvantages of long reaming times and fixations to the bone being processed. Carrying out what are today common muscle-sparing approaches was not possible. Intraoperative changes in the implant position could only be reached by switching to a conventional implantation technique.

Simplest form: procedures for preoperative planning

Most costly form: surgical robots

- More disadvantages than advantages

There followed the so-called navigated operations in which it was possible for the surgeon to perform an intraoperatively "controlled" preparation of the implant site and position with or also without being directly constrained by preoperative planning data. The first systems thus again put into place preoperative CT datasets and planning procedures in which the bone positions were intraoperatively matched in order to ascertain the position of the instruments and implants with the camera system required for navigation. These very elaborate systems were followed by so-called kinematic systems in which the bone positions were captured by the movement of the leg and scanning of bony landmarks by the camera system. This technique with infrared camera systems and infrared transmitters or reflectors on the surgical instruments has become established over the last ten years in knee and hip endoprosthetics.

Navigated operations: intraoperatively controlled preparation of implant site and position

Technique with infrared camera system and infrared transmitters or reflectors on surgical instruments

Meta-analyses of various studies show that through navigation malpositioning in terms of positioning outliers are reduced. This applies in knee endoprosthetics for the position of the axis of the femoral and tibial components and in hip endoprosthetics for the position of the socket. Navigated procedures for soft-tissue balancing in knee endoprosthetics, the optimization of offset, leg length,

Less malpositioning with navigation

Navigated procedure for various tasks in knee and hip endoprosthetics
Disadvantage:
high equipment costs

and range of movement in hip endoprosthetics as well as navigational algorithms and workflows for endoprosthetic revision interventions are also included in this. In conflict with the potential use of navigation is the cost of the equipment. First, routine exposure to the navigation system leads to a non-time-consuming and/or shortened and simplified operation in knee endoprosthetics, and, according to the workflow chosen, to a maximally non-time-consuming hip endoprosthetics implantation of a primary hip endoprosthesis.

In our clinic navigated endoprostheses have been implantedip as a routine intervention since the year 2000 with a proportion of practically 100 % of primary knee endoprosthetics and around 80 % of elective hip endoprosthetics. The use of navigation technology, the surgical procedure and our experiences are described in the following.

7.2 Navigation Technology

Kinematic system:
relevant information in real time on the screen

- Implantation instruments with transmitters
- Recording with video-optical infrared stereo camera system

In a CT-free navigation system, also termed kinematic system (Fig. 7.1), the surgeon receives relevant information in real time on the screen o which schematic images of the bony structures are displayed. For this reason, implantation instruments are equipped with transmitters during the operation that capture the necessary intraoperative recordings with the use of infrared technology. Thus, a video-optical infrared stereo camera system records the position of the transmitter that is found in the recording area. In addition, with the aid of navigation software the site and position of the transmitters to each other and thereby the site and position of the instruments relative to the patient are calculated. For this purpose

Table 7.1: Overview of the suppliers of navigated hip and knee endoprosthesis implantation.

Supplier	Navigation system	Internet
Aesculap	OrthoPlot®	www.orthopilot.de
Brainlab	VectorVision®	www.brainlab.com
Biomet	VectorVision®	www.biomet.de
Johnson & Johnson	VectorVision®	www.jnj.de
DePuy		www.depuy.de
Medtronic	StealthStation®	www.medtronic.com
Smith&Nephew	VectorVision®	www.smith-nephew.de
Stryker	Stryker® System Stryker® eNlite	www.stryker.de
Zimmer	ORTHOsoft® Sesamoid	www.zimmergermany.de

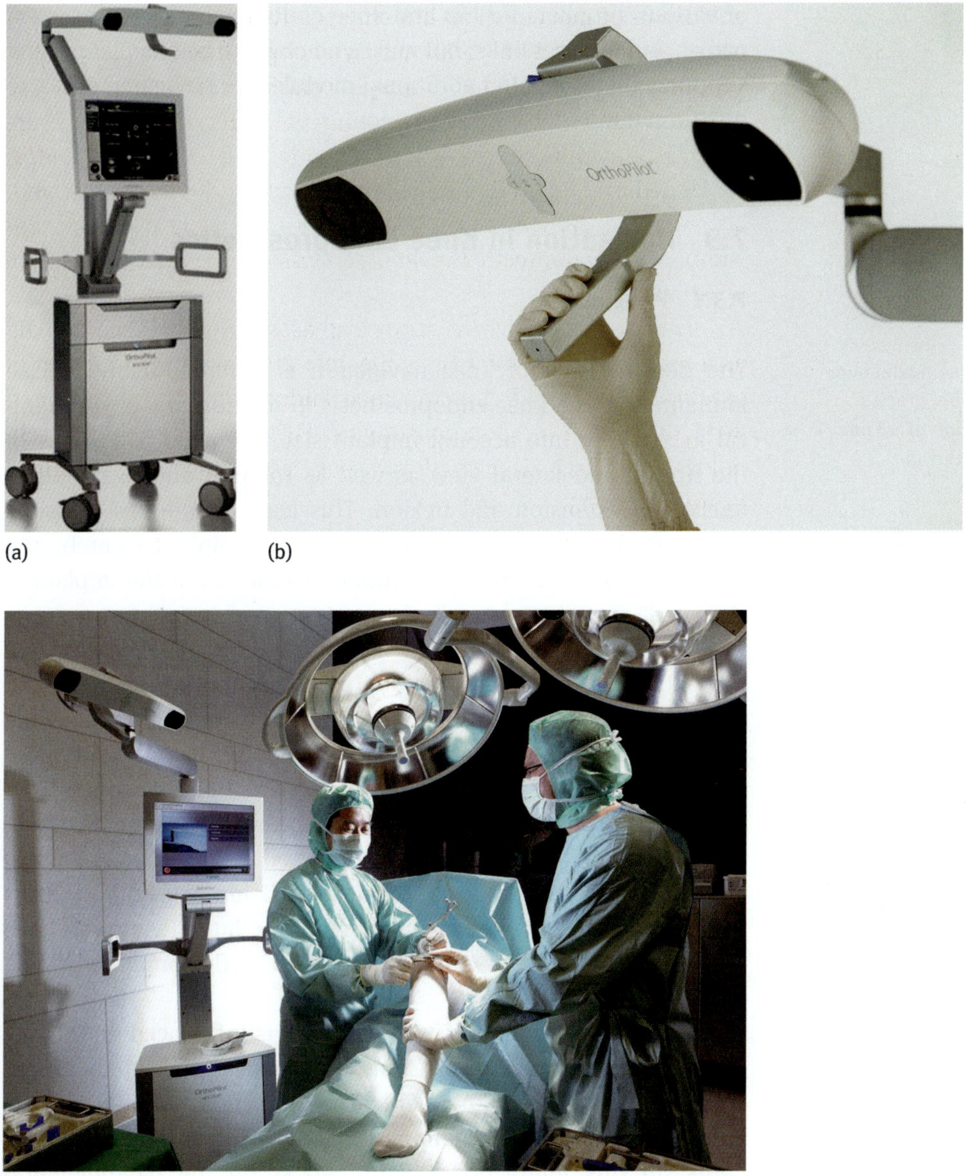

Fig. 7.1: (a) Kinematic Orthopilot navigation system, (b) Orthopilot camera, (c) interaction of navigation/ instrument/patient.

transmitters are fixed to the bone and anatomical landmarks defined during the surgical procedure are picked up by so-called pointers.

▸ Transmitter on bone

Navigation systems are supplied by various manufacturers. For hip and knee endoprosthetics, the endoprosthesis models to be used with them are to be noted. Table 7.1 contains a compilation

Various navigation systems on the market

of various suppliers for hip and knee endoprosthetics with system names and internet links, but makes no claim to be complete. Many suppliers therefore offer additional modules for navigated orthopedic interventions.

7.3 Navigation in Knee Endoprosthetics

7.3.1 Principles

Aim of knee navigation: reproducibly precise implantation of a knee endoprosthesis

The declared aim of knee navigation is a reproducibly precise implantation of a knee endoprosthesis in relation to a 0° mechanical axis taking into account implant size, the axial conditions in the frontal and lateral view as well as rotation and ligamentous tension in extension and flexion. This leads to the best possible and even division of load across the whole implant whereby the overriding aim of increased duration of function of the implant is expected.

Consideration of patient's individual anatomy with the aid of bony landmarks and kinematic data

A particular consideration has found since the beginning of navigation the patient's individual anatomy through recording of specific or several bony landmarks and the recording of kinematic data on hips, knee, and ankles of the patient to be operated upon. A skewed inserted tibial or femoral component or both in the frontal view, can lead to incorrect weight-bearing, i.e., an increased unilateral articulation load with increased risk of material wear, and thus consequently to a premature revision, e.g., due to prosthesis loosening. Skewed components in the lateral view can have movement limitations (with extension and/or flexion deficits) as a consequence.

Influence of the interaction of the femur and tibia due to various factors

The interaction of the femur and tibia is influenced on the one hand by the ligamentous tension of the medial and lateral collateral ligaments and on the other by the right choice of implant size, implant position, and rotational position of the implant components. In this interaction the influences on the patellofemoral mobile bearing also have to be considered.

"Overstuffing" can lead to anterior knee pain

If the position of the femoral components is too anterior, where the anterior shield is above the bone, we speak of so-called "overstuffing." This can in individual cases lead to increased patellar pressure, which the patient expresses as anterior knee pain that is not more narrowly defined.

Notching can produce a breaking point at the femoral bone

If on the other hand the femoral component lies too far dorsally, which is shown through sawing in the anterior area of the cortex, thus, we speak of so-called "notching". In extreme cases such a "notching" can produce a breaking point in the femoral bone. In a postoperative fall incident, a femoral fracture can occur in patients in exactly this position.

Rotational position of the implant influences the course of the patella

The rotational position of the implants influences the course of the patella. Early revisions of knee endoprostheses because of malrotating implant components with patellar problems that can be expressed as partial or complete subluxation of the patella are described.

Lower revision rate with safe zone of ± 3° around the 0° mechanical axis

Movement limitations, obvious axial deviations or significant instability in the course of movement or patellar problems are still difficult to justify to the patient. Even before introduction of the navigated implantation technique, in several fundamental works a so-called "safe zone" of ± 3° around the 0° mechanical axis was defined in which revision rates fell significantly lower than in implantations outside of this zone.

Additional information during implantation of a knee endoprosthesis with the aid of the navigation system

With the aid of a navigation system during implantation of a knee endoprosthesis, depending on the chosen application and the data recorded, the following additional information is obtained:
- Data in degrees on varus and/or valgus orientation for that particular mechanical axis – femur or tibia – in the frontal view
- Data in degrees on the anterior and/or dorsal slope to the mechanical axis in the sagittal view
- Resection levels in mm to the recorded reference points
- Size suggestions on the basis of the recorded data
- Measurement and display of both the intraoperatively measured and the residual extension and flexion spaces in mm in a planning simulation
- In most systems in the tibia-first technique with "soft-tissue management" the possibility of the simulation of all femoral cuts including the positioning of the femoral components in both the anterior–posterior dimension and in relation to internal and/or external rotation

Most navigation systems can determine rotation

The intraoperative orientation to determine the rotational position of the components represents a further challenge, which is why most navigation systems offer several possibilities to determine rotation, e.g., recording of the epicondyles, the Whiteside line, and the dorsal condyle line.

Patient's individual implant site preparation and implantation in stages

Assistance in minimally invasive approaches

The display of data takes place during bone treatment with saws and before implantation of the final implant components. Thus, the patient's individual implant site preparation and implantation is performed in stages. In smaller, minimally invasive incisions and under limited viewing conditions, navigation is of particular assistance and supports the surgeon in the secure placement and alignment of the implant.

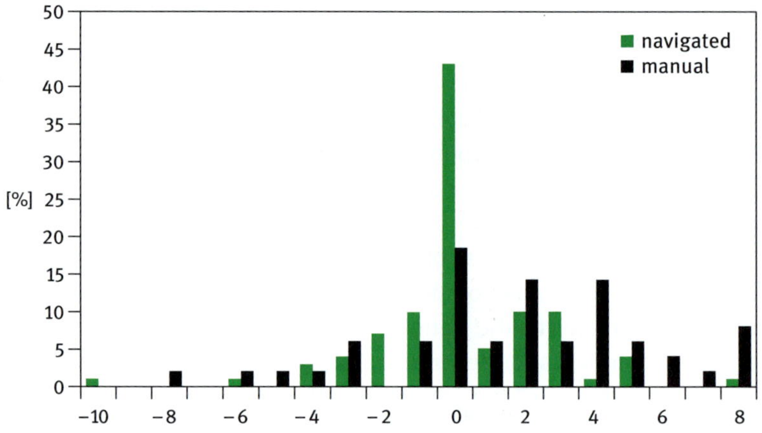

Fig. 7.2: Mechanical axis postoperatively. Distribution of the individual values around the ideal 0° axis (Kiefer et al. 2001).

Reduction of outliers outside the safe zone

Early works and/or studies already showed a significant difference in navigation from the conventional technique, namely, the reduction of outliers outside the defined safe zone of ± 3° varus/valgus (Fig. 7.2).

So far no proof of higher survival rate in the long term with navigated implantation

Risk of malalignment significantly lower with navigation

Proof of plausible consistency after achieving optimal alignment with the best possible distribution of load, lower risk of wear, and thus a reduction of the aseptic loosening even in the long term, achieving a significantly higher survival rate through navigated implantation, could not be provided so far. The exemplary meta-analyses mentioned at the beginning show that the risk of a malalignment > ±3° varus/valgus, which correlates with the risk of early loosening of the implant, is significantly lower with navigation. Fig. 7.3a and b give in the form of forest plots a good overview of the available literature sources that are all in favor of navigation.

7.3.2 Surgical Procedure

Navigation systems in knee endoprosthetics with many different applications

Extent of predominant surgical techniques/software applications. These days, navigations systems in the field of knee endoprosthetics offer a multitude of different applications, that the doctor supports, to implement the best possible implant positioning. These range from applications of purely axial navigation in the "femur-first" technique, via axial navigation in the "tibia-first" technique, up to the "tibia-first" technique with consideration of the soft tissue – so-called "soft-tissue management" – and simulation of the results on a planning screen for the preparation and positioning of the femoral components.

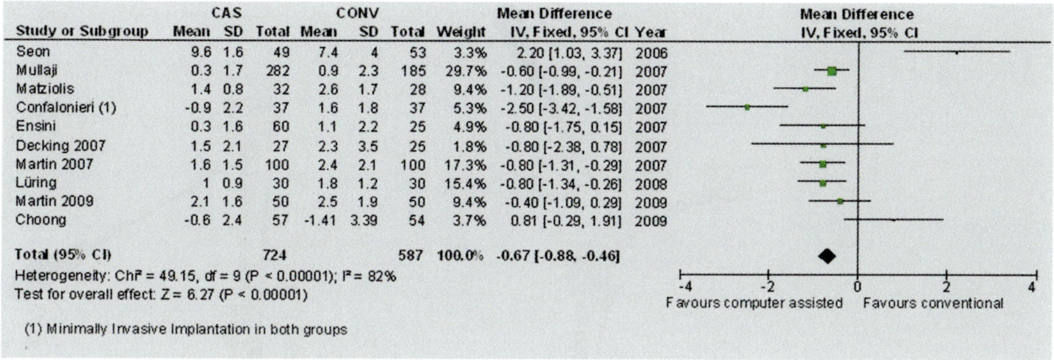

(a)

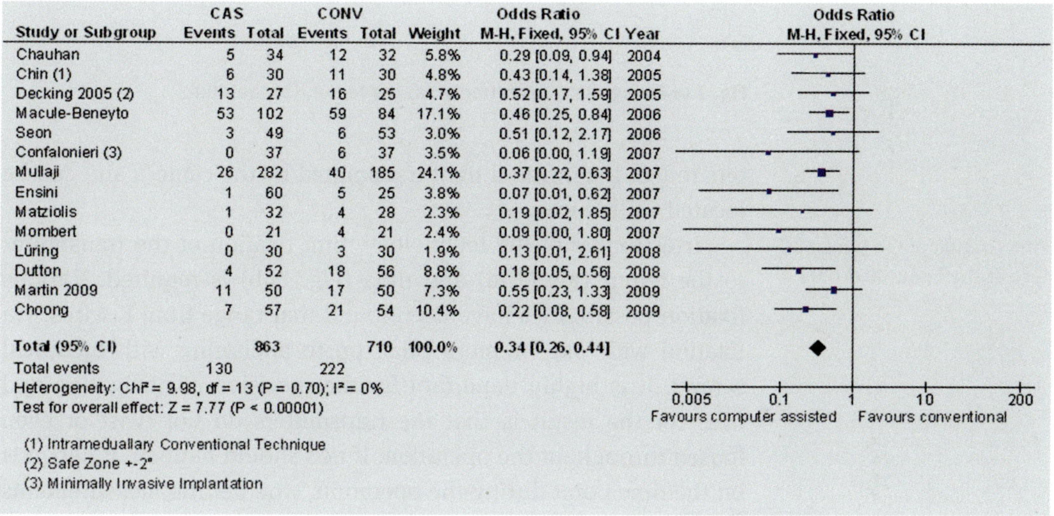

(b)

Fig. 7.3: (a) Alignment (means and standard deviation); (b) number of knee joints with axial deviation of more than 3°.

Preparation for navigated knee surgery. The preparation and positioning of patients do not vary considerably from the conventional technique. When adjusting the side supports a certain freedom of movement in the hip area should be given, to determine the mechanical axis. The sterile covering is almost identical.

> Preparation and positioning as with the conventional technique

Technological aspects. All current navigation systems work with infrared camera systems, which record the movement of three different transmitters, although active and passive transmitters are distinguished. Active transmitters transmit infrared light and therefore require a power supply by cable or batteries. Passive transmit-

> Infrared camera systems with active or passive transmitters

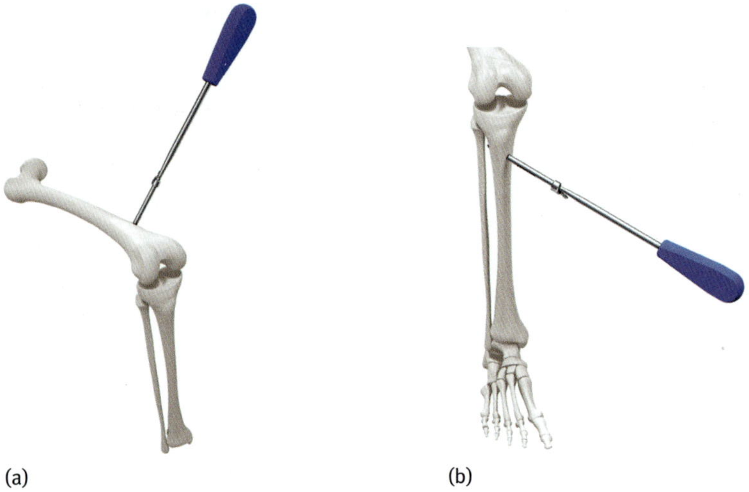

Fig. 7.4: Fixing the transmitter to (a) the femur, (b) the tibia.

ters reflect the infrared light transmitted by the camera and can be located in this way.

Firm fixation of the transmitters at the femur and tibia

Irrespective of the technology, firm fixation of the transmitter to the femur (Fig. 7.4a) and tibia (Fig. 7.4b) is required. Various fixation possibilities have been found that range from K-wires, via fixation with one or more pins, up to anchoring with bicortical screws. It is highly important for the precision of navigation and thus for the result is that the transmitters do not twist or even loosen throughout the operation. If this should happen, it depends on the time point during the operation, whether the measurements can be repeated with reattached transmitters or whether it is necessary to change to the manual technique. After one or more of the transmitters has loosened, the values can no longer be relied upon.

After loosening of the transmitters measurements can no longer be relied upon

Determination of the kinematic hip center to capture the mechanical axis

Capture of the mechanical axis. The capture of the mechanical axis is performed by all navigation systems, even if this can be carried out via various algorithms and anatomical landmarks. To determine the mechanical axis, at the same time, various algorithms and the kinematic hip center and/or center of the femoral head through movement of the femur are determined (Fig. 7.5).

Evaluation of the knee center via landmarks or capture of the kinematic knee center

For the evaluation of the knee center, the medial and lateral dorsal condyle as well as the anterior cortex can be used as examples of bony landmarks. Alternatively or additionally, evaluation via the capture of the kinematic knee center occurs, which for example through flexion, extension, and rotational movement of the leg and thus through the tracing of the movement of the femoral and tibial transmitters (Fig. 7.6).

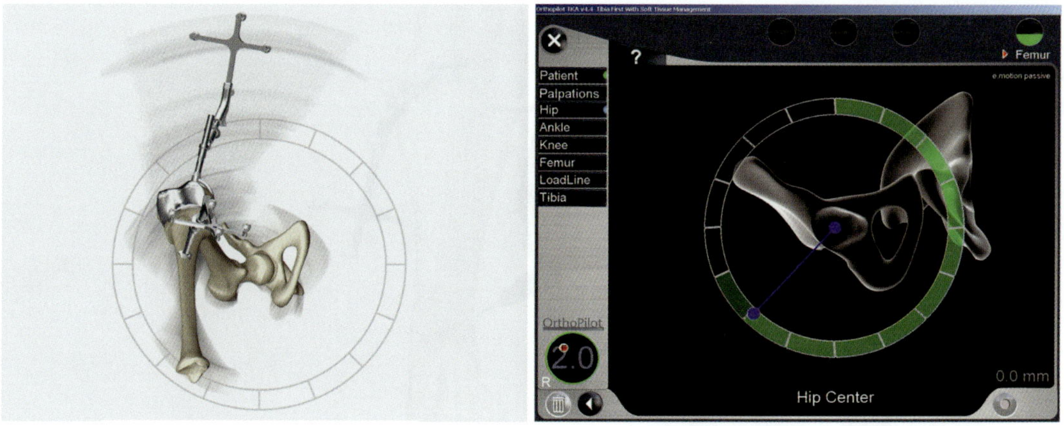

(a) (b)

Fig. 7.5: (a, b) Registration of the hip center.

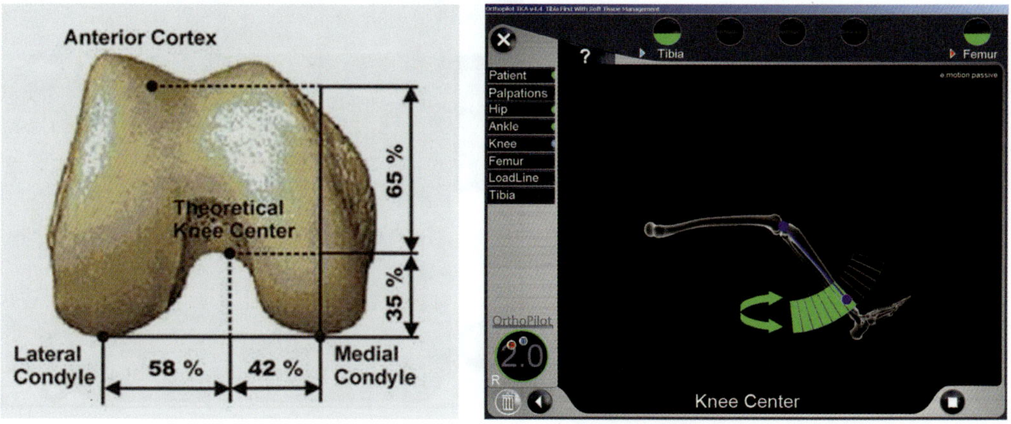

(a) (b)

Fig. 7.6: (a) Theoretical knee center of the femoral side; (b) registration of the knee center (Picard et al. 2007).

To determine the mechanical tibial axis a point recording in the center of the tibial plate is carried out and at the distal end of the tibia, for example, over the recording of the most prominent malleolar points medially and laterally, as well as the recording of an anterior point, the center of the ankle is determined (Fig. 7.7).

Determination of the mechanical tibial axis

Similar to that already described above for the knee center, some systems also offer the possibility of capturing a kinematic center for the ankle by recording the extension and flexion movements of a non-invasive transmitter on the back of the foot in relation to the tibial transmitter (Fig. 7.8).

Capture of the kinematic ankle center

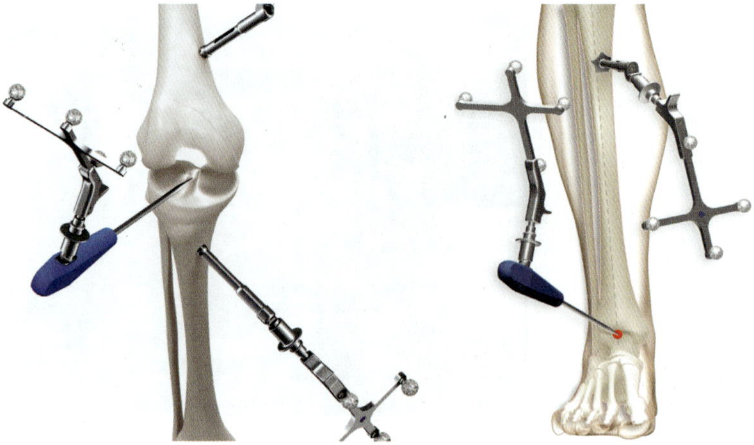

(a) (b)

Fig. 7.7: (a) Determination of the center of the proximal tibia; (b) registration of the ventral ankle point.

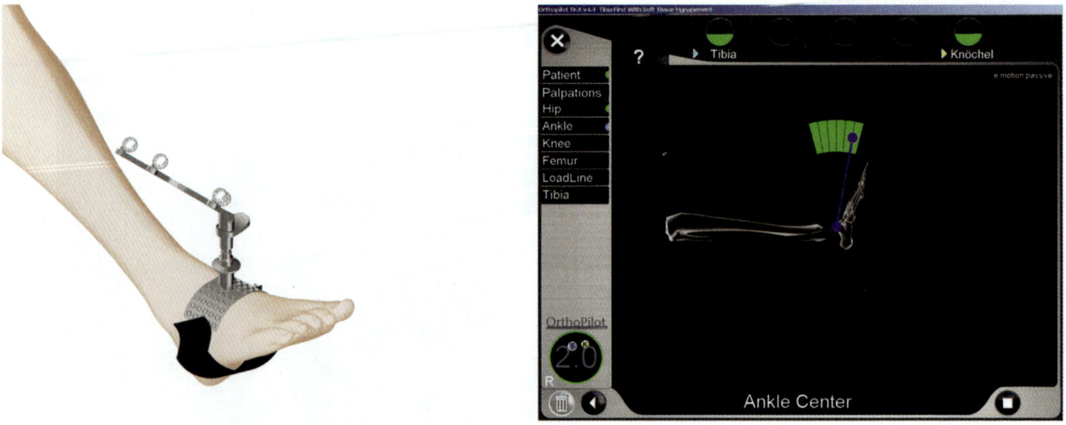

(a) (b)

Fig. 7.8: (a, b) Determination of the ankle center.

Visualization of the leg axis present

After determining the ankle center the capture of the mechanical tibial axis is completed and the navigation system can visualize for the doctor information about the present patient's leg axis (Fig. 7.9). The degree data are identified as the difference between the mechanical femoral and the mechanical tibial axis. Thus, a valgus or varus leg position can be quantified and possibly any extension or flexion deficits present can be verified by degree data

Further anatomical landmarks as reference points

Registration of anatomical landmarks. Further anatomical landmarks needed for the precise determination of size of the femoral component or also to note the incision level for the alignment of

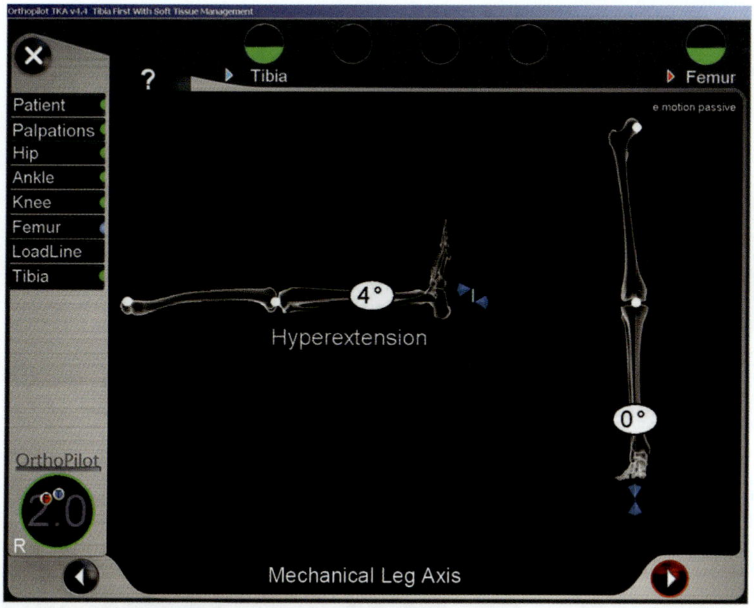

Fig. 7.9: Visualization of the mechanical leg axis.

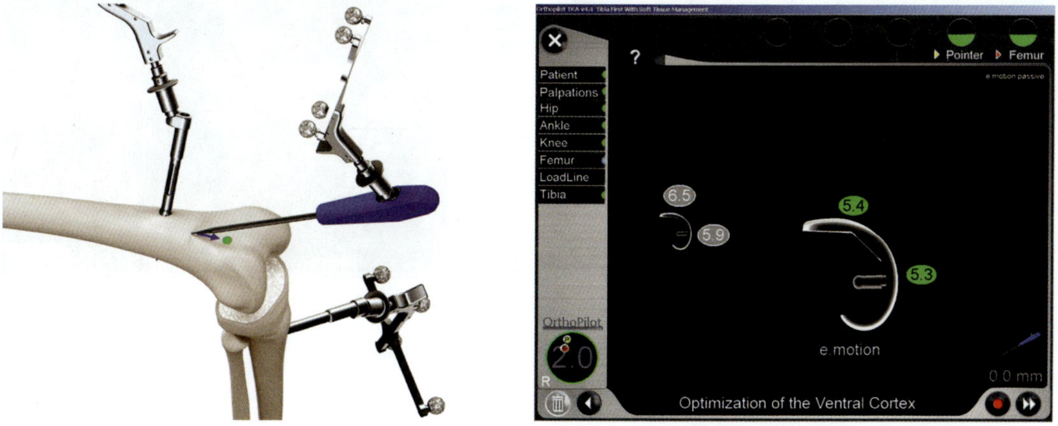

(a) (b)

Fig. 7.10: (a, b) Optimization of the ventral cortex.

the saw blocks (Fig. 7.10). On the registration of reference points and/or reference levels both for the tibia incision and for the distal femoral resection the precise incision level at these points can be noted (Fig. 7.11).

In which sequence proximal tibial incision and distal femoral incision are carried out depends – as described above – on the preference of the surgical technique used, although both techniques (femur-first or tibia-first) have their advantages and disadvantages.

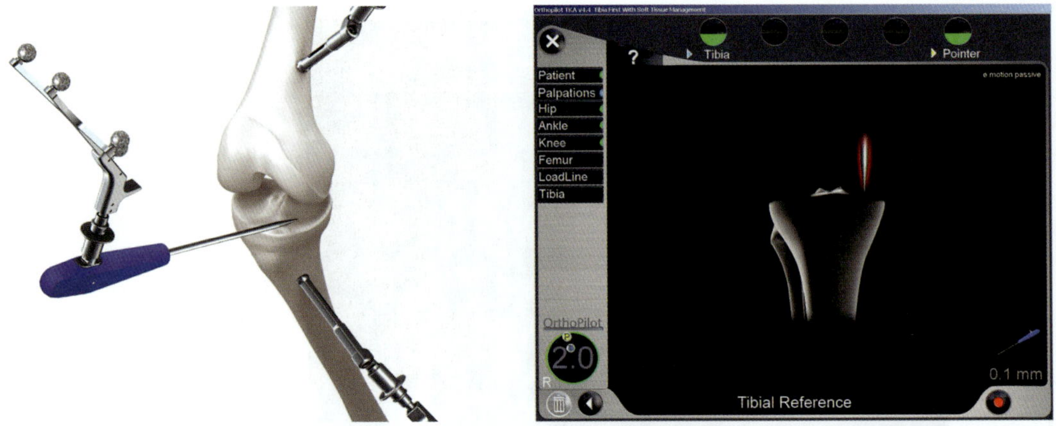

(a) (b)

Fig. 7.11: (a, b) Palpation of tibial reference points.

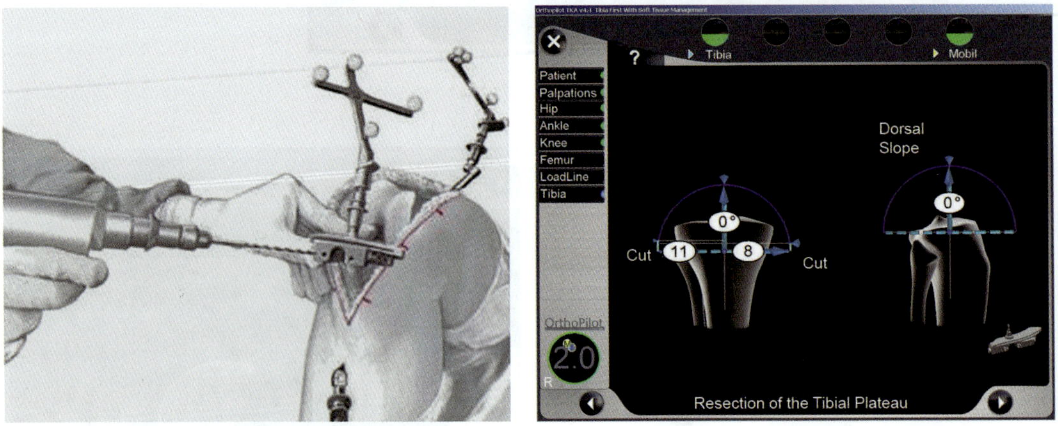

(a) (b)

Fig. 7.12: (a) Alignment of the tibial saw block; (b) resection of the tibial plateau (Magin MN 2010).

Precise alignment of the saw template

Performance of resections. For the alignment of the saw template for both incisions: it can now be carried out precisely in the frontal and sagittal views and under control of the incision level according to the previous recorded references (Fig. 7.12). The incisions can then be carried out as desired.

Ligament instability the main reason for early revisions

Measurement of the ligamentous tension. In 2001 Fehring et al., after a precise analysis of 440 revised patients after TKA, reported an early revision rate of 50 % within five years after the first operation. At 27 %, instability was the main reason for these revisions. Sharkey et al. also showed that at an early revision rate of 55 % within the first two years after the first operation, instability was

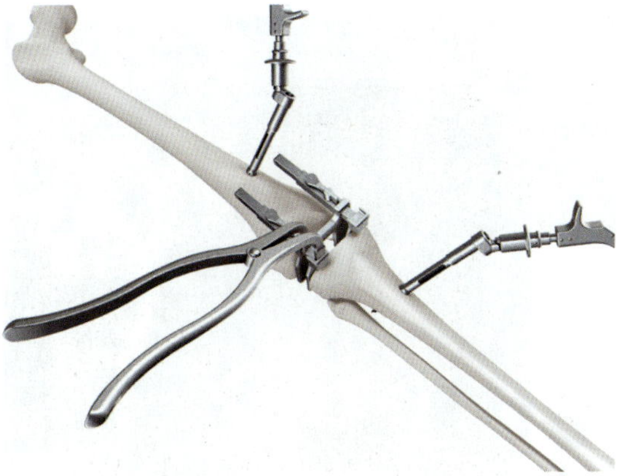

(a)

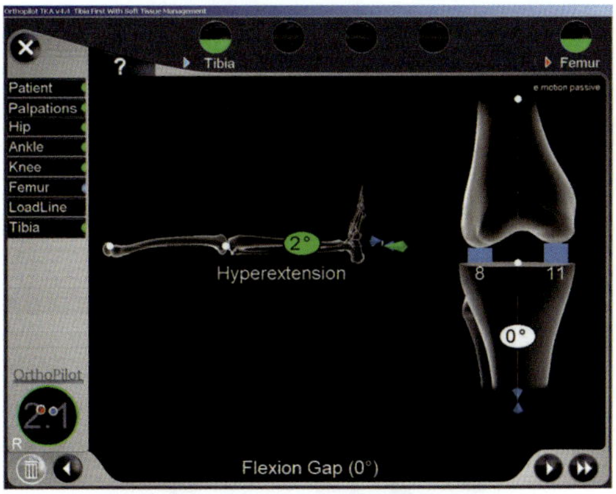

(b)

Fig. 7.13: (a, b) Measurement of the joint space in extension.

also responsible for 21 % of the revision cases. Against this background the measurement of ligamentous tension, the so-called "gap management" or also "soft-tissue management" was accorded a special significance.

Tibia-first technique: determination of the ligamentous tension on insertion of a spreader between tibial and femur

In the tibia-first technique, which is often termed the gap-balancing technique, there is the possibility, depending on the software available, of determining the ligamentous tension via the insertion of a spreader between the tibia and femur (Fig. 7.13). Thus, the spreader is in contact with the resection surface of the tibia and the distal and/or dorsal condyles in the measurement of the flexion gap. For the measurement it is important that spreading is done medially and laterally each with the same force. To ensure this, spreaders that defined the force were developed. If in spreading in extension an axial deviation of 3° or more varus or valgus occurred, often a stepwise release is advisable. After each release step has been carried out a new measurement of the extension gap should be made to control the progress achieved in relation to the axis deviation.

▸ Measurement in extension

Afterward the measurement in flexion (Fig. 7.14) is made. In 90° flexion the spreader is again inserted and if possible with the same force medially and laterally and/or spread over a spreader that defines the force. The values of the measured space in flexion can influence a.p. positioning, rotation, and the size of the femoral components as well as the level of the PE inlay.

▸ Measurement in flexion

The effectiveness of soft-tissue management with the help of a navigation system could already be shown in individual studies. Lampe et al. say that navigation systems thus allow precise positioning of the implant and balancing of the soft tissues in the minimally invasive technique without raising the complication rate.

Soft-tissue management for soft-tissue balancing

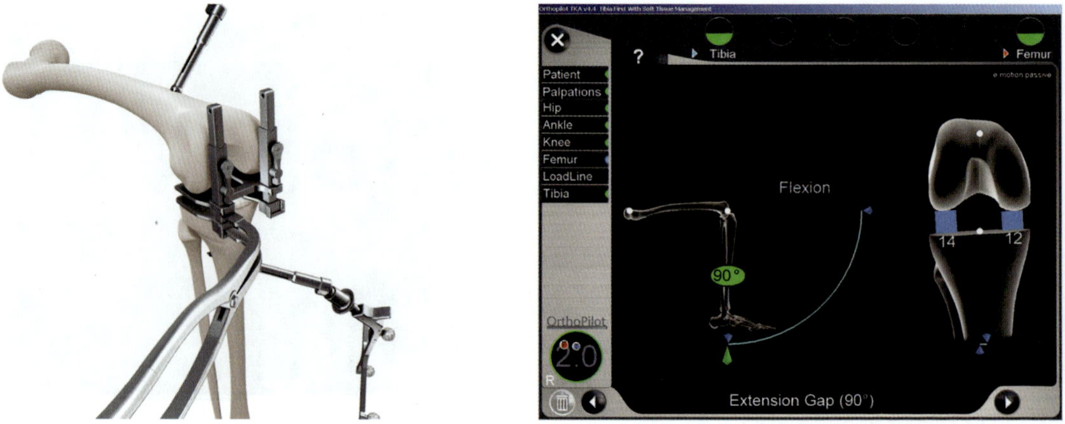

(a) (b)

Fig. 7.14: (a, b) Measurement of the joint space in flexion.

Seon et al. report that navigation with soft-tissue management leads to well-balanced knees with superior anterior–posterior laxity.

Femoral planning. After successful tibial resection and measurement of gaps in extension and flexion, most of the navigation systems available offer the possibility of planning the upcoming incisions at the femur and to simulate the result of this planning (Fig.

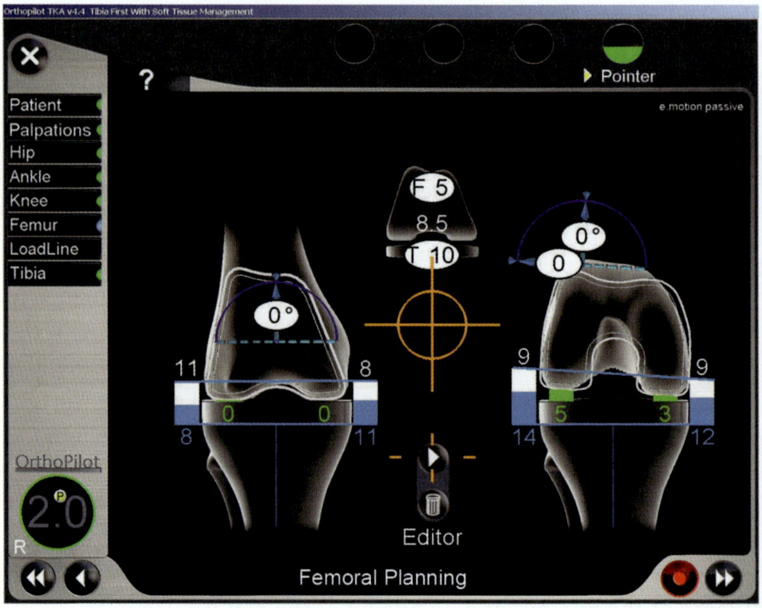

Fig. 7.15: Femoral planning.

7.15). The following parameters can therefore be introduced into femoral planning:

- Varus/valgus orientation
- Distal incision level
- Size of the femoral component
- Level of the polyethylene inlay
- A.p. positioning of the femoral component
- Rotational position of the component
- In some systems even the slope/extension/flexion position of the femoral component in the sagittal view

Planning of the upcoming incisions at the femur

After planning of the position of the femur and all femoral incisions is completed, the alignment of the saw block follows.

Registration of the real incision values for checking purposes

Verification of the results and plausibility checking. After each incision the majority of navigation systems offer for checking purposes the registration of real incision values in order to carry out checks of the planned values from the saw guide position (Fig. 7.16). Consequently, corrections can be made at any time.

Plausibility checks in the navigation workflow

Doctor retains control during the whole operation

At several time points during the navigation workflow, plausibility checking can be carried out on the one hand, by measurements and comparison with preoperative X-rays; on the other, through the use of manual examination instruments. The assignment of robotic systems also appears to be significant. The doctor remains in the final analysis the decision-maker and also makes the incisions himself, i.e., he always retains control during the whole surgical procedure.

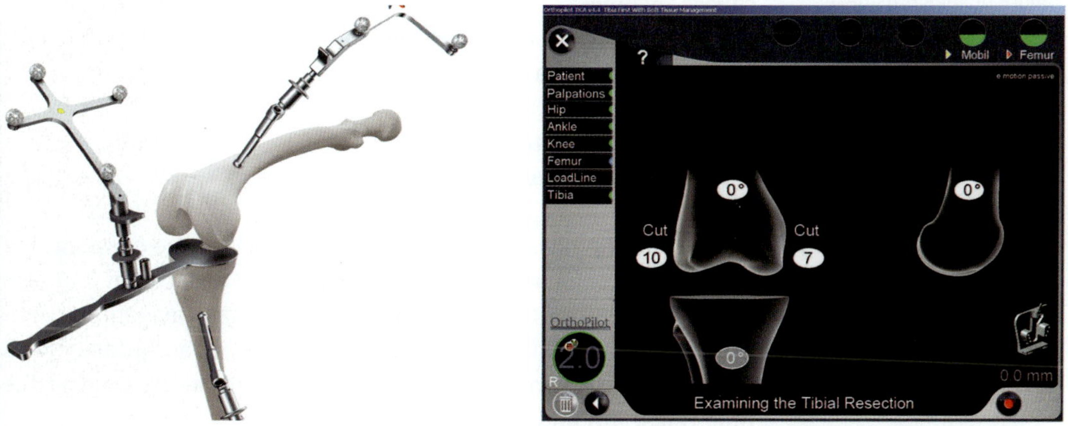

(a) (b)

Fig. 7.16: (a, b) Examining the tibial resection.

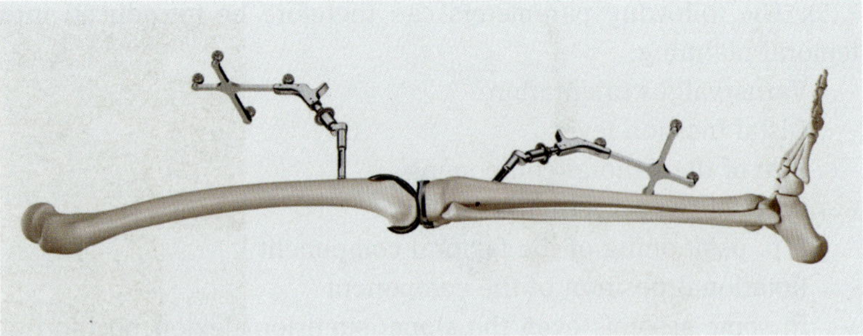

Fig. 7.17: Mechanical axis.

Implantation with manual instruments

Testing via the display of the mechanical axis

Implantation and testing. After preparation of the femur and tibia for the implants is complete, which is mainly carried out with manual instruments, an initial examination with test components and lastly with the final implant, also takes place. The testing takes place via display of the mechanical axis on the monitor. This recording can be directly related to the mechanical axis registered at the beginning of the intervention (Fig. 7.17).

7.3.3 Special Aspects

Navigation always more important in knee revision interventions

Because of the constantly rising number of revision interventions today and in the future of navigation, a more and more important and significant role falls to this field of knee endoprosthetics. Here, the navigation can make a very important additional contribution. Navigated knee revision interventions are still at the beginning of development and are certain to increase in significance.

Reasons for high rates of failure of knee prostheses

The reasons for high failure rates are multifaceted, but frequent causes include:

- Shifting, above all, proximalization of the joint line with resulting patella baja
- Defective axial alignment
- Malrotation of the implant
- Bad balance from extension to flexion gap

Features of the revision software

Features of the revision software are in particular the possibility of joint line planning and much more, its precise dislocation, but also the preparation of the lengthening stems under navigational control parallel to the mechanical axis and/or in accordance with available offset variants of the implant system being used at the time (Figs. 7.18 and 7.19).

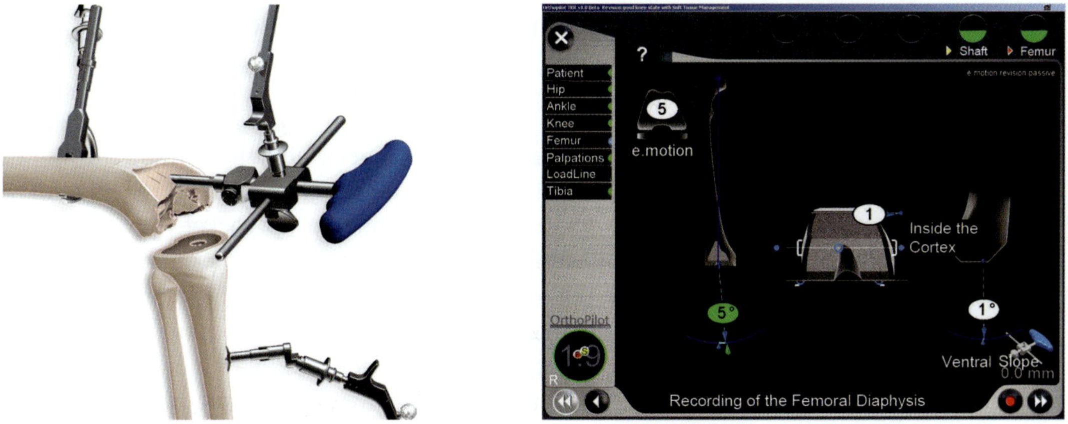

(a) (b)

Fig. 7.18: (a, b) Recording of the femoral diaphysis.

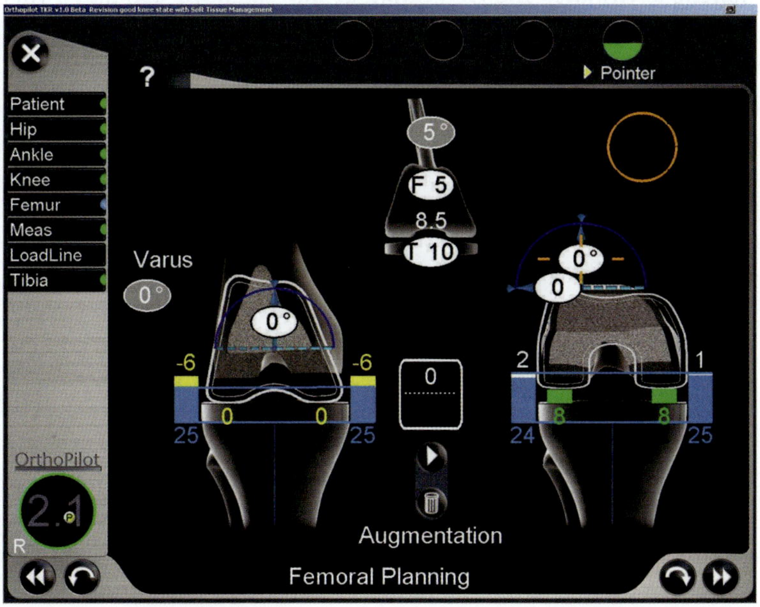

Fig. 7.19: Femoral planning.

7.4 Navigation in Hip Endoprosthetics

7.4.1 Principles

Aim of navigated hip implantation: reliable orientation points for alignment

Navigated implantation of an artificial hip joint follows the aim of communicating to the surgeon during the operation reliable orientation points in the alignment of the hip socket, the prosthesis stems, and adjustment of the socket and stem position, taking into consideration the anatomical and patient-specific situation.

Complications with the alignment of the hip socket and the stem

In the alignment of the hip socket a component that is implanted too steeply or too flat can lead to an increased articulation load or movement limitation with implant impingement or even to a joint luxation. The same applies to the socket anteversion positioning in the case of anteversion that is too strong or even retroversion positioning. The interaction of stem and socket component determines the free range of movement of the hip. Thus, stem torsion and socket anteversion have a functional relationship. A reduction in the femoral offset has a significant effect on the joint stability and the range of movement; the resulting significant increase in leg length is these days hard to justify to the patient.

Safe zone: radiological socket inclination 40° ± 10°, socket anteversion 15° ± 10°

Regarding the position of the socket, in a classical work on the influence of socket position and dislocation behavior a "safe zone" was also defined if the socket lies within a radiological socket inclination of 40° ± 10° and a socket anteversion of 15° ± 10°.

Total values of anteversion and antetorsion important for optimal range of movement

With regard to the optimal range of movement there is a relationship between the total values of the socket anteversion and the femoral antetorsion of the prosthesis stem, which was reported by Widmer to have a value of 37.3° – socket anteversion + 0.7 × stem antetorsion. The anteversion and antetorsion values are in no way easy for the surgeon to determine intraoperatively and they can also deviate preoperatively in the planning or postoperatively from standard X-rays.

Intraoperative orientation to the socket position via anatomical landmarks

The intraoperative orientation to the socket position occurs at the anatomical landmarks of the acetabulum and the use of mechanical positioning guide, the use of which is routine; however, its precision is limited by the variability of the patient's position. In particular, the intraoperative evaluation and quantification of the femoral torsion position is a challenge even for an experienced surgeon.

Aim: prevention of early joint instability

An artificial hip joint therefore offers great variability of implant positions, which in interaction are not always easy to evaluate in combination. Furthermore, as the artificial hip replacement has a high success rate, cases with early joint instability are frustrating if this could have been prevented by another implant position.

It should also be noted that surgical approaches of anterolateral and directly anterior are generally feasible with muscle-sparing and therefore increase the muscular joint stabilization. With the muscle sparing posterior approach the risk of subluxation has also been lowered by reconstructive techniques in which the capsule is sutured. The use of larger prosthesis heads, 0.036 m instead of 0.028 m or 0.032 m, has contributed to this. The latter, however, cannot hide the fact that larger heads increase the edge loads of the socket component and therefore the principles of good socket positioning remain valid.

Through muscle-sparing approaches an increase in the muscular joint stabilization

Gandhi showed in a meta-analysis that a navigated implantation leads to a reproducible socket position. Unfortunately, there are no works that prove improved long-term results. Only a few works are concerned with the navigation of the stem and socket component and could reproducibly establish leg length adjustment or offset reconstruction.

Navigation:
- Reproducible socket position
- No improved long-term results

When the use of a navigation system is decided, it is established that the conflict with individual and patient-specific implant

With navigation, more intensive conflict with implant treatment

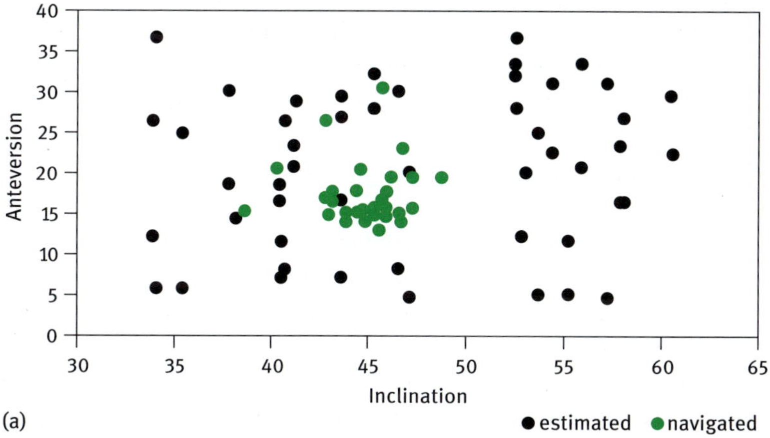

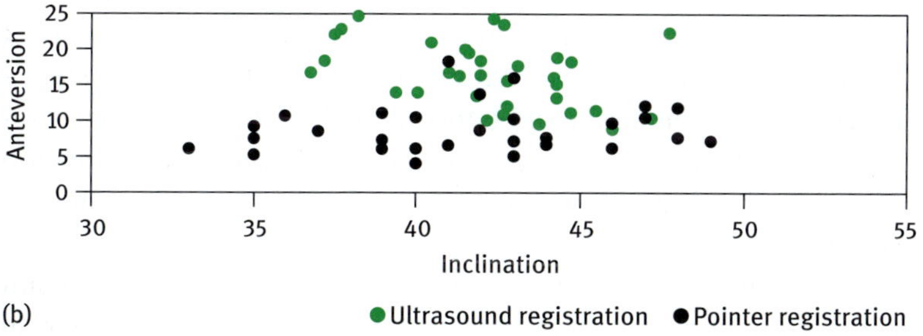

Fig. 7.20: (a) Socket positioning with and without navigation (Lazovic 2006); (b) socket positioning navigates with pointers and ultrasound referencing (Kiefer 2007).

treatment becomes significantly more intensive than if the only the surgeon's feeling and experience are relied upon (Fig. 7.20). The training for endoprosthetic implantation is also different for the surgeon.

Intraoperative data on socket and stem positioning via navigation software

On the monitor of the navigation system the surgeon receives intraoperative data on socket and stem positioning irrespective of the navigational software chosen:
- Socket inclination
- Socket anteversion
- Change in leg length
- Change in offset
- Range of movement
- Stem antetorsion

Patient-specific implant site preparation and implantation in stages

Help with minimally invasive procedures

The data display occurs during work on the bone with acetabulum reamers or stem rasps and before implantation of the final implant components. Thus, patient-specific implant site preparation and implantation is performed in stages. Navigation is a good aid, particularly in smaller, minimally invasive incision guidance and under limited visual conditions, and supports the surgeon in the secure placement and alignment of the implant.

7.4.2 Surgical Process

Navigated implantation of the socket component most frequent

Fixation of a reference transmitter to the spina iliaca anterior superior

Socket navigation. The navigated implantation of the socket components is the most frequently applied technique that can be combined with further parameters for stem implantation, depending on the software. So that the navigation system recognizes the position of the pelvis, stable fixation of a reference transmitter to the spina iliaca anterior superior is necessary for the whole duration of navigation. This is done on the ipsilateral side of the hip to be operated on with a 0.01-m-long stab incision around 0.03 m posterior to the ipsilateral anterior spina iliaca superior (ASIS). Into this, a suitable retaining screw is put in, onto which the pelvis reference transmitter is then fitted. The transmitter is aligned in the direction of the camera position (Fig. 7.21). All of the following images are shown for a patient in supine position. For the features of the lateral position, please refer to Section 7.4.3.

Precise calculation of inclination and anteversion angle of the socket over precise registration of bony landmarks at the pelvis

A requirement for a precise calculation of the inclination and anteversion angle of the socket is a precise registration of bone landmarks in the pelvis. In the socket navigation the entry level of the pelvis forms the reference level for the inclination and anteversion angle of the socket. The registration of the entry level of the

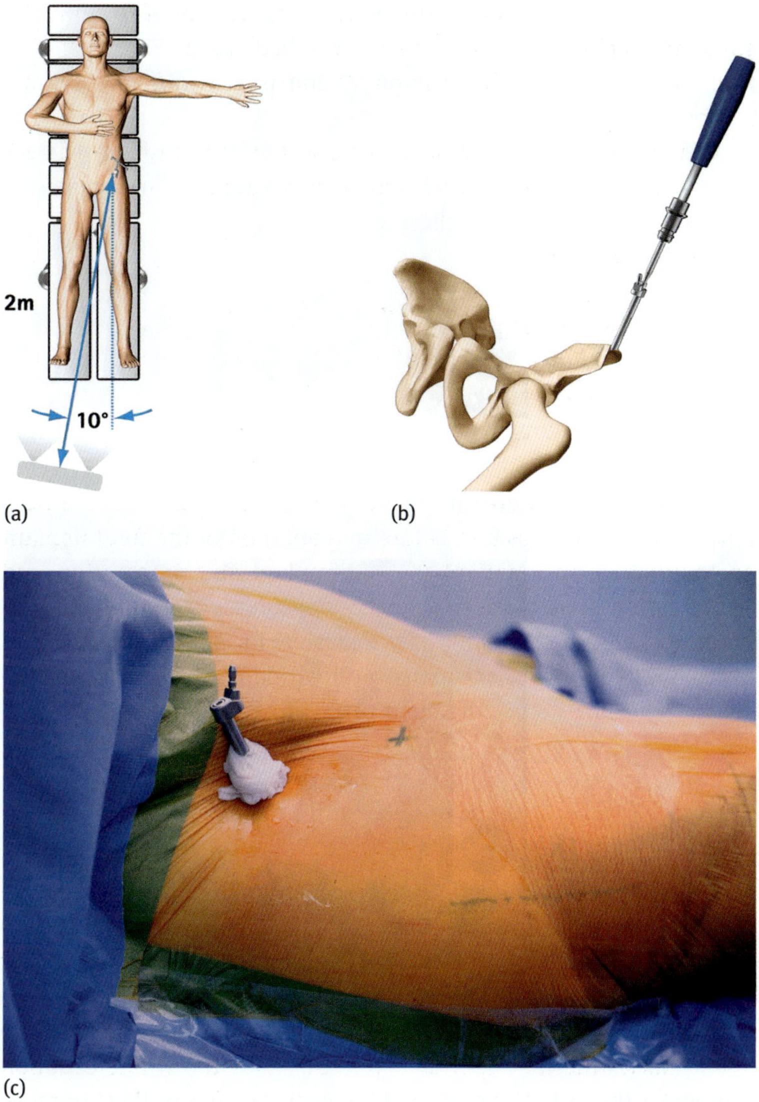

Fig. 7.21: (a) Patient positioning in supine position with placement of the navigation system. (b, c) Percutaneous fixation of a screw at the ipsilateral ASIS for the pelvic transmitter.

pelvis is carried out percutaneously by palpation of both the anterior spinae iliacae superior and the symphysis with a pointer (Fig. 7.22a, c). To enable this, the thickness of the surgical coverage of the spinae iliacae and the symphysis must be consistent. In addition, the surgeon should push aside the subcutaneous fatty layers over the landmarks during palpation. It has been proven that the fatty layers at the spinae iliacae can be pushed from lateral to medial and to take the ledge of bone between two fingers. At the

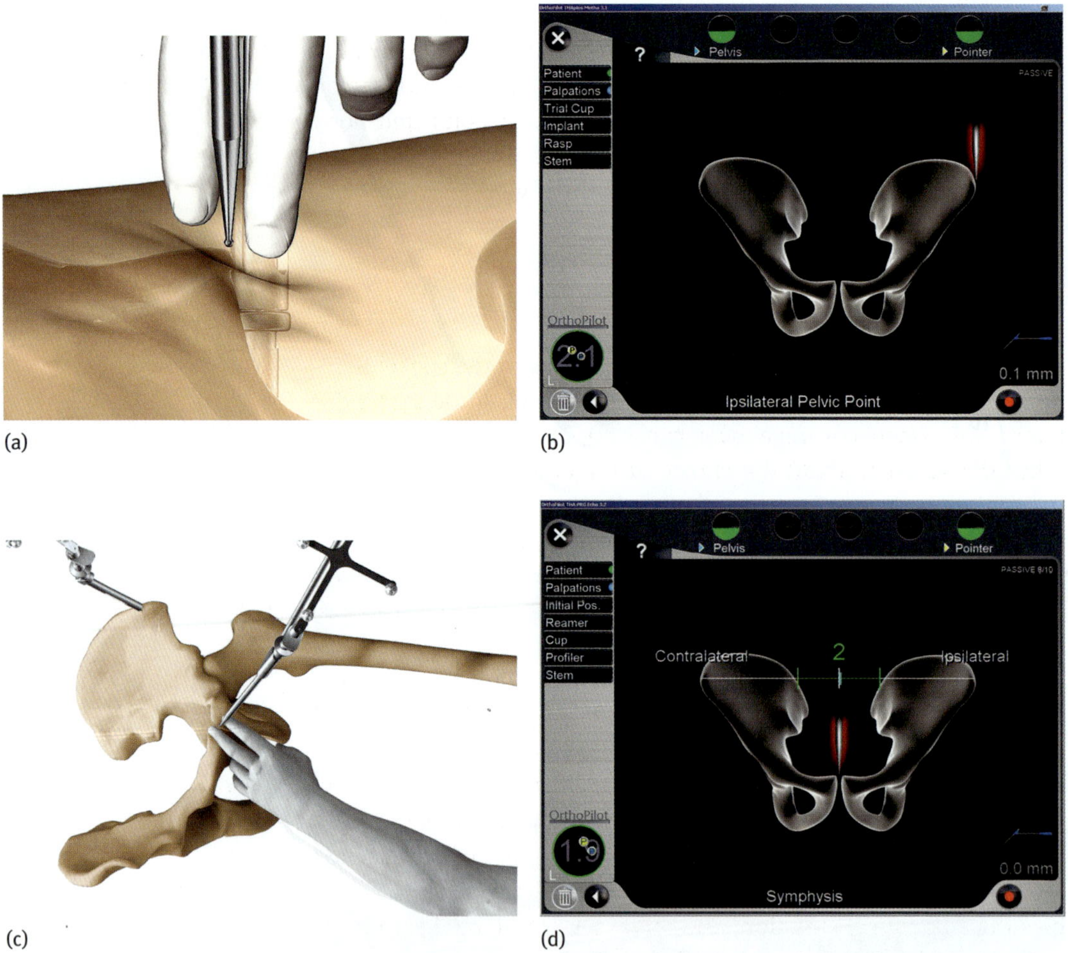

Fig. 7.22: (a, c) Percutaneous palpation of the anterior spina iliaca superior and the pelvic symphysis and referencing with a pointer. (b, d) Corresponding pictures on the monitor of the navigation workflow.

symphysis the fatty layers should be pushed from caudal to cranial. The registration sequence is displayed by the navigation system in the workflow on the monitor (Fig. 7.22b, d).

Determination of the socket inclination angle

The socket inclination angle arises from the straight lines that are defined by the palpation of both anterior spinae iliacae superior. It varies by the landmarks being pushed cranially or caudally. The palpation of the ASIS must therefore be carried out symmetrically (e.g., both points from cranial to caudal). The precision of the registration and the inclination values arise from the deviation from the palpated ASIS position.

Inclination precision:

± 10 mm = ± 1.5°

± 20 mm = 3.0°

The anteversion angle is dependent up on tilting the level, which arises from palpation of all three landmarks, although the level of the symphysis point has the greatest influence on the anteversion angle. With the growing space between palpated point and bony level (corresponds to the thickness of the tissue layer), the anteversion angle displayed on the navigation system gets smaller.

Determination of the anteversion angle

Anteversion precision:

± 0.01 m = –4.0°

± 0.02 m = –12.0°

This means in practice a "more precise" display of the socket inclination and usually less display of the anteversion through the different soft-tissue coverage over the symphysis. As the surgeon takes the decision about the choice of the anteversion position of the socket, he can define the value of the socket implantation and thereby be responsive to the individual situation of the patient.

More precise display of the socket inclination, less display of anteversion

In principle it is also possible to carry out pelvis registration with an ultrasound probe. This method is still new; it shows a more precise evaluation of the anteversion position. The inclination values were not significantly improved, which is an argument in favor of the very good accuracy of the pointer registration described above.

Pelvis registration possible with ultrasound probe

After referencing of the pelvis the position of the acetabulum is also referenced. The methods for this are dependent on the navigation system used. The most frequently used referencing is carried out through a navigated test socket, with which the surgeon examines the anatomical situation, and about which the navigation system obtained a first value of the hip centre and at the same time displayed the inclination and anteversion positioning of the test socket (Fig. 7.23a). With these values it should be considered that at this time point the socket bearing has not yet been reamed.

Referencing of the acetab ulum position, e.g., via navigated test socket

In addition, it is possible to palpate bony points in the acetabulum with a pointer, e.g., the deepest places of the fossa acetabuli, to display or limit the reaming depth, or points on the edge of the socket, in order to input the patient-specific information on the acetabular anatomy into the navigation system.

Palpation of bony points in the acetabulum

Afterward the navigated preparation of the acetabulum begins with reaming. On the monitor, the angles for inclination and anteversion relative to the pelvis entry level are thus displayed (Fig. 7.23b, c). The angle data are helpful for the orientation of the reaming direction and control of the navigation data. In the screenshot shown (Fig. 7.23c) the surgeon receives additional information on the reaming depth (red scale) as well as the three-dimensional shift of the hip centre cranially, medially as well as anterior/posterior in

Navigated preparation of the acetabulum with reaming

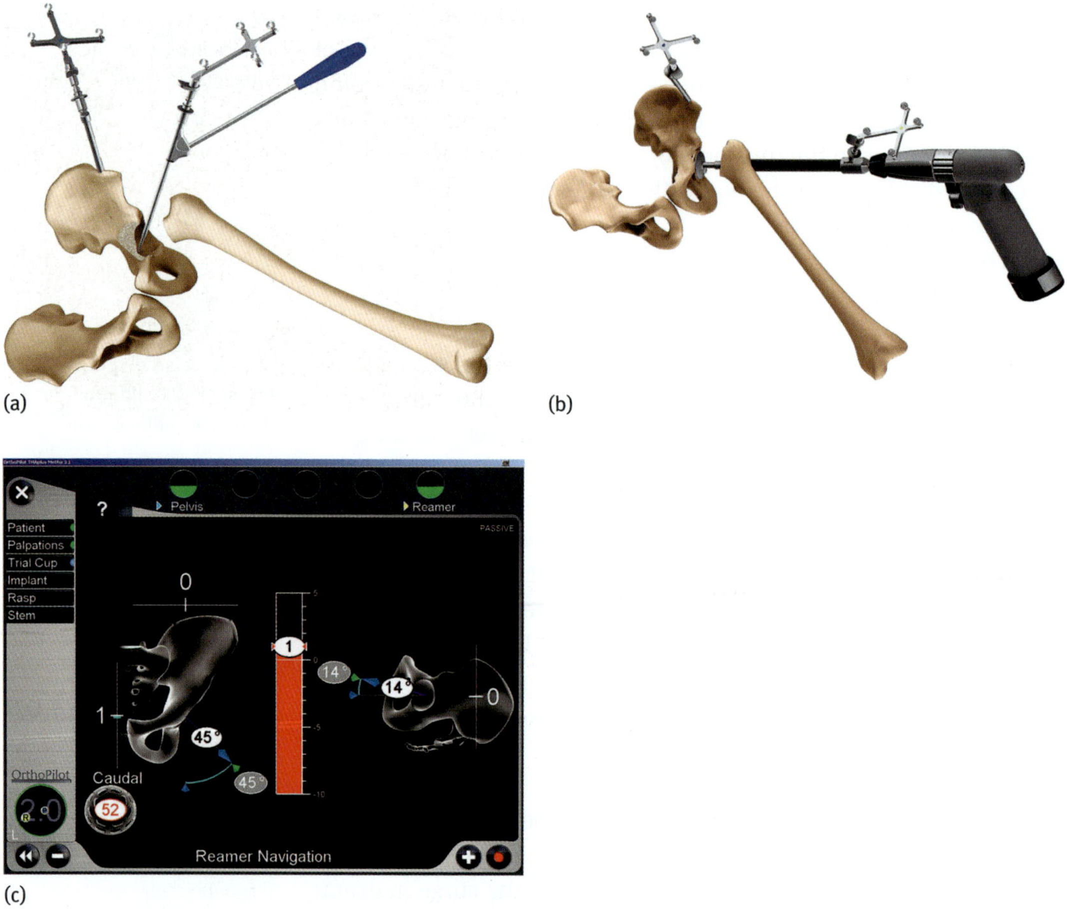

Fig. 7.23: (a) Insertion of a navigated test socket for determination of the joint center and control of the anatomical alignment of the acetabulum. (b) Navigated reaming of the acetabulum. (c) Example of the navigation screen during navigated reaming.

millimeter values. Two values provided in gray on the monitor reflect the starting point of the acetabulum for inclination and anteversion recorded by the test socket. In this way, the new center of the socket can be prepared in accordance with the preoperative planning.

Top aim: secure fixation of the socket implant

The secure fixation of the socket implant remains the top aim with the navigation-supported process as it is with the conventional surgical technique. Therefore, attention should be paid to the system-specific characteristics of the socket implant in the preparation of the implant site.

Navigation system shows and saves final inclination and anteversion values

At insertion of the final socket implant the navigation system again shows the final inclination and anteversion values and saves in a form that is dependent on the navigation system the data produced during implant site preparation and socket implantation

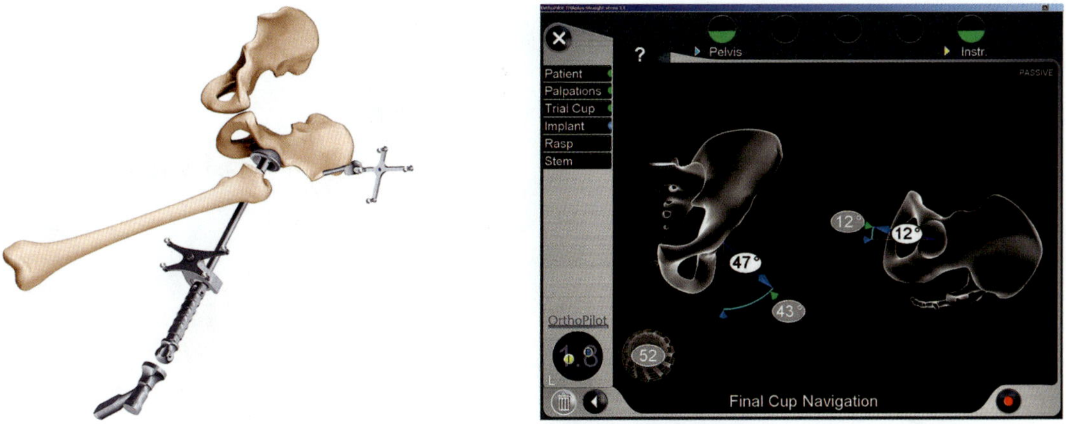

(a) (b)

Fig. 7.24: (a) Navigated insertion of the acetabular socket component. (b) Monitor display of socket inclination and socket anteversion.

(Fig. 7.24). These can be used for the surgical and treatment documentation.

Implantation in usual sequence

The implantation of the prosthesis stem follows. This process is consistent with the usual implantation sequence of a hip endoprosthesis. Details of the procedures by which the prosthesis stem is first planted are to be found in Section 7.4.3.

Stem navigation with or without reference transmitters at the femur

Stem navigation. For the navigation of the stem component there are workflows with and without fixation of transmitters to the femur. This plays an important role in that without transmitter reference a lower amount of data can be captured, but the lack of transmitter reference simplifies the surgical process.

Fixation of a reference transmitter at the femur

Fixation of a reference transmitter to the femur is usually more difficult to carry out juxta-articularly than distally in the area of the femoral condyles. The distal reference is less precise owing to the greater distance to the hip joint and is not supported by any navigation system. If a femoral transmitter is fitted, this must occur at the beginning of the operation, i.e., before the navigated implantation of the socket component described at the start.

Femur and pelvis references allow very precise determination of all parameters of hip endoprosthesis

Femur and pelvis references allow the very precise determination of all the parameters of hip endoprosthesis, such as offset, leg length, stem antetorsion, and range of movement (Fig. 7.25). The new center of the hip and rotatory alignment of the femur are influenced both by implantation of the socket and by the stem. Offset and leg length can be displayed thereby as absolute or relative values in terms of deviations due to the implantation of an artificial hip joint. Data on the range of movement can be effected by simulation of the navigation system and by the display of real movements. Owing to pathological

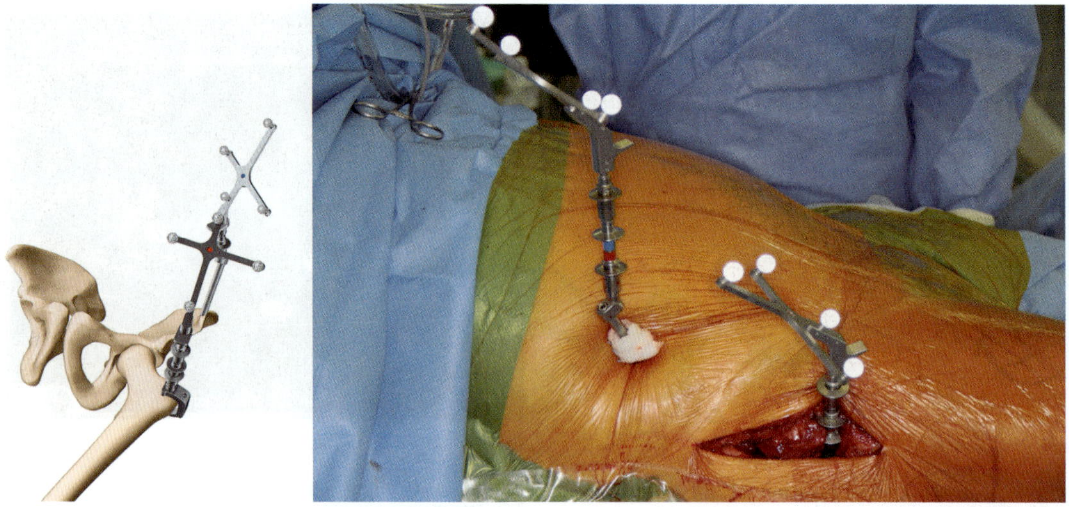

(a) (b)

Fig. 7.25: Pelvic transmitter and juxta-articular femoral transmitter reference schematically (a) and in situ (b).

changes to the hip joint, however, the surgeon must decide which values he would like to achieve and to what extent the implant system used enables the implementation of hip joint reconstruction.

By referencing absolute indication of values for antetorsion of the femoral component

In pelvis and femur referencing, the surgeon receives during the femoral preparation an absolute indication of values for the natural and the implant-induced (and/or previously prepared by rasping) antetorsion of the femoral component. The surgeon can already obtain this value, which is usually referenced on the dorsal knee condyle line, by opening the medullary cavity with a box chisel, and consequently change or retain with navigated rasping during the femoral preparation.

Femoral implant allows which femoral antetorsion can be achieved

Which value can be implemented for the femoral antetorsion by the implant also depends on the femoral implant. Resurfacing, for example, allows no changes; a straight stem can limit the rotator position owing to anatomical conditions or lead to a relative retrotorsion. A short stem inserted over the femoral neck or an anatomically formed standard stem triggers a usually positive antetorsion in the joint that also closely approximates the natural conditions. Stem systems with modular necks adapters permit a basically freer choice and approach to the femoral joint center.

Values calculated and simulated by the navigation system

After insertion of the stem rasp the surgeon receives on the monitor a real indication of the femoral torsion and simulated data on the range of movement, the maximal flexion and change in leg length and offset for all available head sizes. After implantation of the stem component these values can be accessed again before the final implantation of the head components (Fig. 7.26).

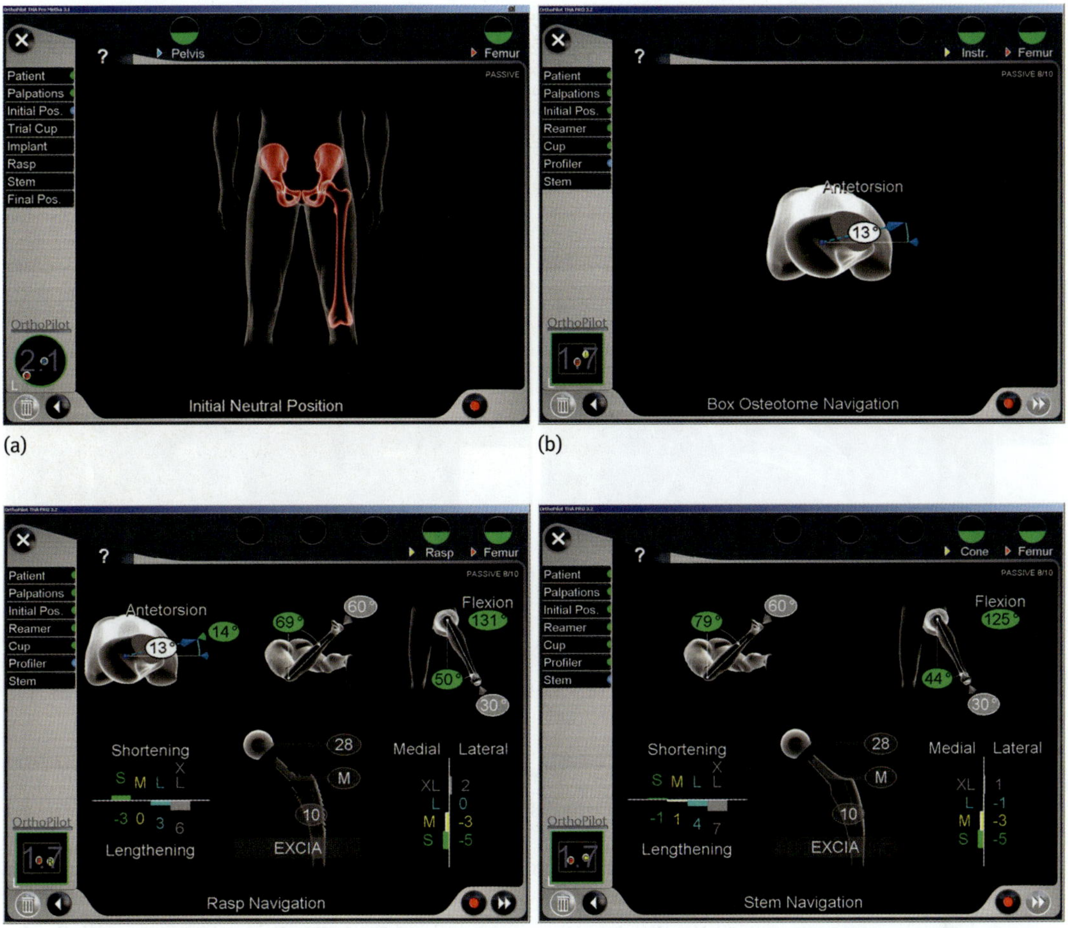

(a) (b) (c) (d)

Fig. 7.26: Stem navigation: starting position (a), display of femoral antetorsion before rasping (b), simulation after rasping (c), and result after implantation (d).

There is also the possibility of navigating the femoral offset and the leg length of a hip endoprosthesis treatment without implantation of a femoral reference transmitter. This is an advantage in minimally invasive surgical approaches. This is followed by the registration of the femoral reference by the same recording of a patellar and a trochanter point (Fig. 7.27). The leg must be brought into 90° flexion. Both points should each have been marked previously, as they have to be palpated again in the navigation sequence. The point at the trochanter major is the reference for the offset value. Optimally, the trochanter major must be palpated at its most lateral point – indicated by the red shading on the screen. As a possible marker, a cortical screw or a deeper lying notch can be used at the bone surface if required. Over the pal-

Navigation of offset and leg length also possible without femoral transmitter
- Advantage for minimally invasive approaches

- Referencing of patella and trochanter points

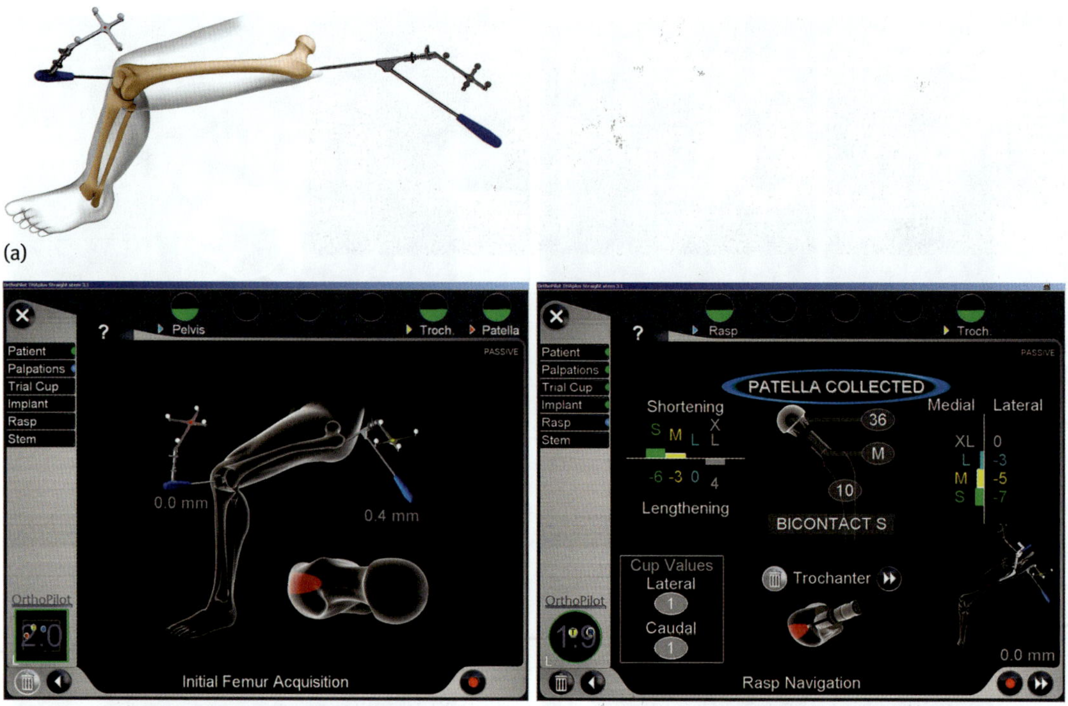

Fig. 7.27: Stem navigation without femoral reference transmitter; femur referencing at the trochanter major and patella (a, b), display of leg length and offset depending on the stem sizes and head components used (c).

pated point at the patella the leg length is referenced. The optimal point usually lies on the patella axially between the lower and middle third and can, for example, be indicated by a sterile peg.

Recognition of the position of the rasp via infrared transmitters in the instrument's hand grip

Patellar point references leg length

Trochanter point references offset

After implantation of the socket component (see Section 7.4.2) the femur is prepared by rasping. The navigation system recognizes the position of the rasp via the infrared transmitter on the hand grip. To determine the leg length and the femoral offset, the points that were imported and marked on the patella and trochanter major at the beginning of the operation are re-imported consecutively, although first the patella is recorded in 90° flexion and afterward the trochanter point. The patellar point references the leg length, the trochanter point the offset. On the screen the surgeon can conduct the choice of stem size and/or rasp size, as well as the head diameter and neck lengths. The effects on leg length and offset are depicted according to the head–neck lengths.

7.4.3 Special Aspects

In principle, a navigated hip endoprosthetic intervention can be carried out in the lateral position. In the lateral position in particu-

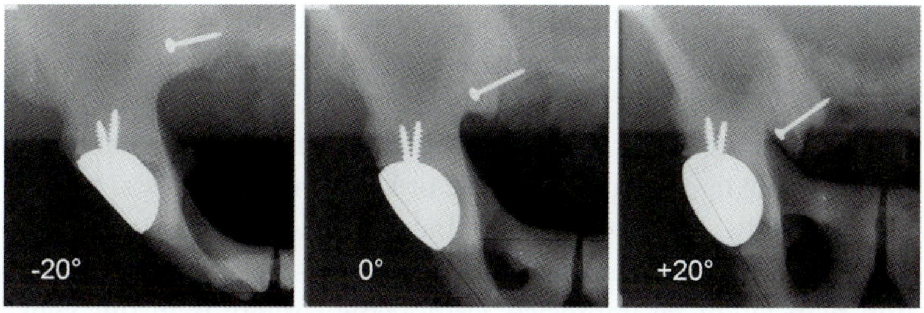

Fig. 7.28: Radiological socket position on the pelvis model with −20°/0°/+20° pelvic tilt.

lar, the orientation in the socket positioning is impeded. In lateral positioning the navigation system is established at the head. A difficulty is the palpation of the contralateral anterior spina iliaca superior, as this is harder to access because of soft tissue, surgical coverage, and padding than when the patient is supine.

Navigated hip endoprosthetic intervention also possible in the lateral position

A further consideration of hip navigation is the so-called pelvic tilt, which influences the radiographic evaluation and real socket position pre-and postoperatively. A pelvic tilt of ± 20° compensates for the anteversion and reduces the inclination of the socket in flexion and increases the anteversion and inclination in extension (Fig. 7.28).

Pelvic tilt influences socket position

Rousseau was able to show in 328 patients with unilateral hip endoprosthesis that the pelvic tilt varies significantly postoperatively. The direction and extent of this variation are thus not predictable. Therefore, the socket position must lie within a narrow target area of a safe zone in order to balance functional tilting of the pelvis.

Pelvic tilt varies considerably postoperatively

Supplementary to the examples described and the processes of the navigated implantation of a hip endoprosthesis, the so-called "stem-first" method is referred to, in which the stem implantation is carried out before the socket implantation. In principle, some navigation systems offer this implant variant in order to implant the socket anteversion onto the femoral stem torsion in a combined anteversion position. Thus, the final implantation of the socket component balances out the limited positioning possibilities of the stem rotation.

Stem-first method: stem implantation before socket implantation

7.5 Outlook

The use of a navigation system for the implantation of hip and knee prostheses improves the reproducibility of the results and the quality of the operation. An influence on the functional results and the durability of the implant has, however, not yet been proven. In

Navigation system:
- Improved reproducibility, quality

- No proof of influence on function, durability
- Expensive, costly

clinical application, the navigation is linked with costs and additional expense. So what are the arguments in favor of the application of navigation technology?

It is required that a surgeon achieves the aim of a reliable and reproducible implantation of a hip or knee endoprosthesis. It is the responsibility of the doctor to define the treatment aim in advance and intraoperatively achieve it as well as possible, even if an operation plan might be imprecise. Orthopedic surgery is in this sense not a "medical art," but a technique with high requirements for safety and efficiency.

Navigation:
- Much more precise, quantitative depiction of the joint anatomy, physiology
- Intraoperative and individual measurement allows individual adaptation

Navigation results in a much more precise, quantitative depiction of the anatomy and physiology of the operated joint. Implant positions at the hip, and ligamentous balance at the knee can be so precisely positioned that instability is often prevented. The intraoperative and individual measurements of the kinematics and the anatomy of the joint and associated soft tissue apparatus allow a very individual adaptation of the prosthetic reconstruction to the patients. With that, one distances oneself from one identical reconstruction "for all," which, particularly for patients with an unusual anatomy, far removed from the average, can lead to difficulties.

- Helps surgeons to learn and perfect joint replacement
- Instrument of quality control and research

Finally, navigation offers an important role in the learning and perfecting of joint replacement for younger, but also for more experienced surgeons. The immediate feedback of the navigation system helps a young surgeon to understand the functioning of the joint and the influence of a practical operative step. In this way, navigation becomes a real instrument of quality control. The precise, navigated measurements can serve as a comparison of new techniques with standard procedures. Navigation is therefore not only an instrument of measurement, but also an instrument of research that has the potential to become the key to future advances in joint endoprosthetics.

References

Brin YS, Nikolaou VS, Joseph L, Zukor DJ, Antoniou J. Imageless computer assisted versus conventional total knee replacement. A Bayesian meta-analysis of 23 comparative studies. Int Orthop 2011;35(3):331–9. Epub 8. 4. 2010.

Fehring TK, Odum S, Griffin WL, Mason JB, Nadaud M. Early failures in total knee arthroplasty. Clin Orthop Relat Res 2001;392:315–8.

Gandhi R, Marchie A, Farrokhyar F, Mahomed N. Computer navigation in total hip replacement: a meta-analysis. Int Orthop 2009;3:593–7.

Harvie P, Sloan K, Beaver RJ. Computer navigation vs conventional total knee arthroplasty: Five-year functional results of a prospective randomized trial. J Arthroplasty 2012;27(5):667–72.

Hasart O, Perka C, Tohtz S. Comparison between pointer-based and ultrasound-based navigation technique in THA using a minimally invasive approach. Orthopedics 2008;31(10 Suppl 1):31–4.

Hetaimish BM, Khan MM, Simunovic N, Al-Harbi HH, Bhandari M, Zalzal PK. Meta-analysis of navigation vs conventional total knee arthroplasty. J Arthroplasty 2012;27(6):1177–82.

Jeffery RS, Morris RW, Denham RA. Coronal alignment after total knee replacement. J Bone Joint Surg Br 1991;73(5):709–14.

Jenny JY, Clemens U, Kohler S, Kiefer H, Konermann W, Miehlke RK. Consistency of implantation of a total knee arthroplasty with a non-imagebased navigation system: a case-control study of 235 cases compared with 235 conventionally implanted prostheses. J Arthroplasty 2005;20(7):832–9.

Kiefer H, Langemeyer D, Schmerwitz U. Computergestützte Navigation in der Knieendoprothetik. European Journal of Trauma 2001;E-Suppl 1: S128–32.

Kiefer H, Othman A. The Orthopilot navigation system for primary bicontact total hip replacement. Z Orthop Unfall 2007;145(Suppl. 1):S49–S52.

Lampe F, Bohlen K, Dries SPM, Sufi-Siavach, Hille H. Accuracy of implant alignment and early results after minimally invasive vs. conventional OrthoPilot-navigated Columbus TKA. Orthopedics 2007;30(10 Suppl): 107–11.

Lazovic D, Kaib N. Results with navigated bicontact total hip arthroplasty. Orthopedics 2005;28(10 Suppl):S1227–33.

Lewinnek GE, Lewis JL, Tarr R, Compere CL, Zimmermann JR. Dislocations after total hip-replacement arthroplasties. J Bone Joint Surg Am 1978;60:217–220.

Magin MN. Computernavigierter Gelenkersatz am Kniegelenk mit dem Orthopilot. Oper Orthop Traumatol 2010;22(1):63–80.

Mainard D. Navigated and nonnavigated total hip arthroplasty: results of two consecutive series using a cementless straight hip stem. Orthopedics 2008;31(10 Suppl 1):22–6.

Moskal JT, Capps SG. Acetabular component positioning in total hip arthroplasty: an evidence-based analysis. Arthroplasty 2011;26(8):1432–7.

Novicoff WM, Saleh KJ, Mihalko WM, Wang X, Knaebel H-P. Primary total knee arthroplasty: a comparison of computer-assisted and manual techniques. Instr Course Lect 2010;2010(59):109–17.

Picard et al. Computer assisted total knee arthroplasty. Berlin: Pro Business GmbH, 2007:286.

Renkawitz T, Schuster T, Grifka J, Kalteis T, Sendtner E. Leg length and offset measures with a pinless femoral reference array during THA. Clin Orthop Relat Res 2010;7:1862–8.

Renkawitz T, Wörner M, Sendtner E, Weber M, Lechler P, Grifka J. Grundlagen und neue Konzepte in der computernavigierten Hüftendoprothetik. Orthopäde 2011;40(12):1095–100.

Rousseau MA, Lazennec JY, Boyer P, Mora N, Gorin M, Catonné Y. Optimization of total hip arthroplasty implantation: is the anterior pelvic plane concept valid? J Arthroplasty 2009;24(1):22–6.

Seon JK, Song EK, Yoon TR, Bae BH, Park SJ, Cho SG. In vivo stability of total knee arthroplasty using a navigation system. International Orthopaedics (SICOT) 2007;31:45–8.

Sharkey PF, Hozack WJ, Rothmann RH, Shastri S, Jacoby SM. Why are total knee artrhoplasties failing today? Clin Orthop Relat Res 2002;404:7–13.

Thielemann FW, Clemens U, Hadjicostas PT. Computer-assisted surgery in revision total knee arthroplasty: early experience with 46 patients. Orthopedics 2007;30(10 Suppl):S132–5.

Wassilew GI, Perka C, Janz V, König C, Asbach P, Hasart O. Use of an ultrasound-based navigation system for an accurate acetabular positioning in total hip arthroplasty: a prospective, randomized, controlled study. Arthroplasty 2012;27(5):687–94.

Widmer KH, Zurfluh B. Compliant positioning of total hip components for optimal range of motion. J Orthop Res 2004;22:815–21.

Appendix: Information on the individual joint prostheses

Joint prosthesis	Shoulder	Hip	Knee	Ankle
Implantations per year	approx. 10,000	approx. 190,000	approx. 160,000	approx. 2,000
Patient satisfaction	Hemiprosthesis: approx. 80 % Total prosthesis: approx. 90 %	approx. 95 %	approx. 85 %	approx. 80 %
Durability	Hemiprosthesis: approx. 83 % after 10 years Total prosthesis: approx. 97 % after 10 years	approx. 90 % after 15 years	approx. 90 % after 15 years	62–95 % after 10 years
Indications	– Primary omarthrosis – Post-traumatic omarthrosis – Avascular humeral head necrosis – Rheumatic arthritis – Instability arthrosis – Defect arthropathy	Dual-head prosthesis: – Osteoporosis-induced femoral neck fracture in older patients – Femoral head necrosis in younger patients Resurfacing (McMinn): – Coxarthrosis in younger, active patients without significant deformity of the joint structures Thrust plate prosthesis: – Coxarthrosis of the "young," active patients with normal bone metabolism and regular morphology of the hip joint	– Gonarthrosis Sled prosthesis: – Isolated medial or lateral joint destruction with intact ligaments and extensive physiological axial conditions Unconstrained bicondylar resurfacing: – Advanced pangonarthrosis with sufficient ligamentous stability owing to intact collateral ligaments Semi-constrained prosthesis: – Pangonarthrosis with insufficiency of the collateral ligaments	– Secondary, post-traumatic arthrosis – Rheumatoid arthritis – Primary arthrosis (rare)

Joint prosthesis	Shoulder	Hip	Knee	Ankle
			Hinged prosthesis: – Gonarthrosis with chronic ligamentous instability – Marked malalignments und contractures – Revision endoprosthetics Modular implants, special prostheses: – Revision endoprosthetics – Oncological orthopaedics Patellofemoral prostheses: – Isolated symptomatic retropatellar arthrosis	
Contraindications, general	– Florid local or system infections – Recent infection in the operation field – General cardiovascular contraindications	– Florid local or systemic infections – General cardiovascular contraindications – Vascular disorders	– Acute or chronic infections of the knee joint – Skin lesions in the area of the operating field – Ulcus cruris – Thrombosis – Nail bed infections – Vascular disorders	– General cardiovascular contraindications – Clinically significant arterial circulatory disorders – Florid or recent infections in the operating field – Systemic infections
Contraindications, special	– Insufficient bone socket in the proximal humerus or in the cavitas glenoidalis – Bad bone quality, e.g., osteoporosis – Neurological diseases such as myopathies, neurogenic arthropathy – Septic arthritis	Dual head prosthesis: – Acetabulum fracture – Protrusion coxarthrosis Resurfacing (McMinn): – Secondary coxarthrosis in dysplasia – Manifest osteoporosis – Coxa vara	Sled prosthesis: – Insufficiency of the anterior/posterior cruciate ligaments – Relative: arthrotic changes of the femoropatellar joint	– High-grade, movement-limiting arthrosis of the upper ankle – Unreconstructable ligamentous insufficiency – Extensive bone and soft-tissue defects after previous operations – Lack of patient compliance – Charcot foot, relevant neurological diseases

Joint prosthesis	Shoulder	Hip	Knee	Ankle
		– Bone cysts in the femoral neck – Femoral head necrosis – Relative: BMI, previous osteosynthesis of the affected hip joint Thrust plate prosthesis: – Osteoporotic femoral neck fracture		– Uncorrectable malalignments – Talar necrosis with defects of the talar dome larger than 50 % – Vigorous physical performance requirements (work, sport)
Cemented/ cementless fixation	– Cemented technique currently standard – Older patients: usually cemented implantation – Younger patients: usually cementless implantation	– Cemented technique currently standard – Cemented implantation – main indication: the older patient with osteoporosis and lower bone density – Cementless endoprosthesis in biologically younger patients with normal bone density measurements	Cemented technique gold standard in the fixation of resurfacing prostheses	Cementless implant fixation has prevailed
Complications	General complications: – Thrombosis/embolism – Postoperative hematoma – Vascular and nerve injury – Wound healing disorders Special complications: – Prosthesis loosening – Glenohumeral instability – Infections	General complications: – Thrombosis/embolism – Postoperative hematoma – Vascular and nerve injury – Wound healing disorders Special complications: – Heterotopic ossification – Impingement – Fractures	General complications: – Thrombosis/embolism – Postoperative hematoma – Vascular and nerve injury – Wound healing disorders Special complications: – Polyethylene wear/aseptic loosening – Ligamentous instabilities	General complications: – Thrombosis/embolism – Postoperative hematoma – Vascular and nerve injury – Wound healing disorders Special complications: – Impingement – Inlay dysfunction – Fractures

Joint prosthesis	Shoulder	Hip	Knee	Ankle
	– Intraoperative periprosthetic fracture – Postoperative periprosthetic fracture – Neurological complications – Postoperative rupture of the rotator cuff Specific complication of the inverse shoulder prosthesis: – “Scapular notching”	– Aseptic loosening – Prosthesis infections	– Prosthesis infections – Anterior knee pain/ patellofemoral pain – Movement deficit/ arthrofibrosis – Injuries of the extensor mechanism – Patellar luxation – Heterotopic ossification – Periprosthetic fractures	– Aseptic loosening – Prosthesis infections – Malalignment/dislocation
Length of hospitalization	5–8 days	Approx. 14 days	5–14 days	10 days
Costs (DRG)	6,000–10,000 €	7,000–13,000 €	5,000–15,000 €	7,500–8,000 €
Revision rate	Hemiprosthesis: approx. 10 % Total prosthesis: approx. 6 %	Approx. 3 %	Approx. 3 % in 2 years p.o.	Approx. 10–20 % in 5 years p.o.
Rehabilitation	– Immobilization in Gilchrist bandage for four weeks – 1st–14th p.o. days: passive shoulder joint mobilization – 3rd–6th p.o. week: development of passive and beginning of active joint movement – 7th–12th p.o. week: development of active joint movement and muscular strengthening – From 13th p.o. week: return to physical work and sport, muscular strengthening, movement exercises	– Early aftercare during the postoperative stationary stay – Follow-up treatment in a rehab clinic or ambulant rehab provision – Ambulant late rehabilitation under care of the resident consultant	– Early aftercare during the postoperative stationary stay – Follow-up treatment in a rehab clinic or ambulant rehab provision – Ambulant late rehabilitation under care of the resident consultant	– From 1st p.o. day passive, then active physiotherapeutic exercise treatment – On 8th p.o. day walker orthosis – Orthosis for 4–6 weeks (X-ray check) – After removal of the orthosis stationary, partially stationary or ambulant rehabilitation provision

Joint prosthesis	Shoulder	Hip	Knee	Ankle
Duration of follow-up treatment	Approx. 3 weeks stationary; afterward further ambulant treatment; Aim 12th week: Painless adduction and retroversion	Approx. 3 weeks; until individually optimal gait pattern achieved with full weight-bearing	Approx. 2–3 weeks	Standardized medication combinations for around 5 months
Follow-up checks	3 months, 6 months, 12 months postoperatively, after that, yearly	Directly postoperatively, 3 months, 6 months, 12 months	1 year, 3 years, 5 years, 10 years postoperatively	6 weeks, 6 months, 12 months
Occupational exertion	– Activities with light to medium loading – If possible no work above the head	– Activities with light to medium loading – Avoidance of frequent squatting positions – Elimination of falling hazards on ladders and scaffolding – If possible avoidance of slippery floors – Avoidance of effects of whole-body vibration	– Activities with light to medium loading – Avoidance of frequent squatting positions – Elimination of falling hazards on ladders and scaffolding – If possible avoidance of slippery floors – Avoidance of effects of whole-body vibration – Avoidance of frequently ascending stairs	– Activities with light to medium loading
Sport	Recommended: – Hiking, walking, jogging, cycling, swimming, aquajogging, physical therapy Conditionally recommended: – Fitness training, regulated strengthening exercises, riding, golf, bowling, skiing, athletics, rowing, sailing	Recommended: – In principle the sport that was practiced before the hip surgery – Sports with rhythmic cyclical movement sequences (e.g., strolling, hiking, walking, Nordic walking, cycling) – Swimming: crawl stroke for the legs up to at least six months after the	Recommended: – In principle the sport that was practiced before the knee surgery – Walking and/or hiking – Cycling (ergometer) – Swimming with crawl or paddle movements With consideration of preventive measures:	Recommended: – Swimming – Hiking – Cycling – Golf – Skiing Banned: – Combat and contact sports – Stop and go disciplines

Joint prosthesis	Shoulder	Hip	Knee	Ankle
	Not recommended: – Tennis, badminton, volleyball, training, football, climbing, mountain biking Banned: – Martial arts, sprinting, bodybuilding	intervention, in addition breaststroke movements – Cross-country skiing (if the patients was trained) – With limitations tennis, gold (straight drive without forceful twisting) Problematic and not recommended: – Contact sports (e.g., football) – Racket sports with fast stop and go mechanisms (squash, badminton) – Sports with axial impact due to frequent jumping – Sports with a slip hazard – Sports in which there is a recognizable danger of luxation because of adversarial contact	– Cross-country skiing – Doubles tennis – Hill walking – Golf Conditionally: – Riding – Bowling – Rowing – (Ballroom) dancing Problematic and not recommended: – Sports that are connected to jerky movements, stopping and twisting movements, extensive adduction and peak loads (e.g., squash, basketball, handball, volleyball, singles tennis on hard courts, alpine skiing)	
Impending infection	If an infection is secondary, i.e., with the help of clinical signs, it can be attempted after less than two weeks to retain this prosthesis. An ultrasound of the joint is immediately carried out, in order to detect fluid build-up and if necessary obtain a spectrum of pathogens by puncture after sending to a microbiology department. Furthermore, immediate rehospitalization and/or stationary treatment; if necessary radical surgical debridement and accompanying high-dose systemic therapy with quinolones, e.g., levofloxacin and rifampicin, for three to six months. If necessary after obtaining an antibiogram, change to the suggested antibiotic			

Index